skullinary delights

Recipes to tickle your funny bone!

Compiled & Edited by
Beth Coltoff Koren

Koren Publications, Inc.

Copyright ©2006 by Beth Coltoff Koren and Tedd Koren, D.C.

All rights reserved. No part of this publication may be reproduced, stored in a retrieval system, or transmitted, in any form or by any means, electronic, mechanical, photocopying, recording, or otherwise, without the prior written permission of the publisher. Printed in the United States of America.

Koren Publications, Inc. • 800-537-3001 • www.korenpublications.com

ISBN: 0-9768255-1-1

For Barbara
Fairy Godmother Extraordinaire

and

for Seth, Shayna and Tedd
who inspire me always to be
the best I can be.

Acknowledgements

My idea for this cookbook would be only that if not for the generous, creative input of a number of people who took the idea to reality.

Several Koren Publications employees, especially Stefani Parino and Robin Skoglund, laughed and laughed as they suggested the names for many of the recipes in this book. From there, Barbara Lipschutz, gourmet chef, shared her love of food by creating the actual recipes.

My husband, Tedd, has been enthusiastic about this project from the beginning, encouraging me along the way. In addition, he contributed the educational comments that accompany each recipe as well as the essay on humor and healing. Teri Duff has shared only a small portion of her vast knowledge in the essay on nutrition and the many choices we make daily about what we eat and how to nourish ourselves toward optimal health. And graphic designer Kim Harding has endowed the book with her tasteful eye and her spirited playfulness.

I am grateful to each of them.

Contents

Introduction 11
Humor and Healing 13

Recipes

Breakfasts

ROMelette with Canadian Bacon 19
Slipped Disc Pancakes with Rotator Cuff Links 20
Western States Omelette 21
Koren Fritters 22
Thomps on Toast 23
Mabel Syrup 24

Hors d'oeuvres and Snacks

Spine-akopita 27
Hip Chips 28
Bone Crackers 29
Lillard Liver Pate 30
Life Party Mix 31
Flesia Pizza 32
Bird Barge 34

Spreads, Sauces and Dips

Tedd's Spread 37
Subloxated Cream Cheese Spread 38
Orthodips 39
Cranialberry Sauce 40
Manipulated Mangoes 41

Salads

Sid's Caesar 45
Hearts of Palmer Salad 46
Regenerated Sprouts 47
Radiculitis Salad 48
Lettuce Adjust You Salad 49

Sandwiches

Luxation Sub 53
Chronic Club 54

Axis 55
Knuckle Sandwich 56
The Rondberger or the Peterson Patty 57
The American Chiropractor Hot Dog 58

Soups and Stews

Lumbar Jack Soup 61
Gonstead Gumbo 62
Lambago Stew 63
Cartilegume Soup..64
Parker 'n' Beans 65
B. J.'s X-ray Consommé 66
Quack Soup 67
Koren Chowder 68

Cheeses and Pastas

Pasta Verdebra 71
Gouda-justment Soufflé 72
Spiney Lobster and Linguine 73
Ruptured Rigatoni 74
Curves and Whey 75
Spinal Spiral Pasta and Peppers 76
Tennis Elbows 77

Meats

Van Rumpt Roast 81
Misaligned Meatloaf 82
Short Leg of Lamb 83
Carver's Delight 84
Tender Ribs 85
Ribley Riblets 86
The Nerve of Ewe 87
Massaged Flank Steak 88

Poultry

Duck á lo'range of Motion 91
Chicken Hips..92
Bruised Celery Ribs with Chicken 93
Knee Jerk Chili...94
Chicken Fingers with Arthrices Stuffing....................................95

Seafood

Dorsal Morsels 99
Sacral Mackerel 100
Pulled Mussels 101
Loxyx Coccyx 102
Gillet Fillets 103
Carp á la Tunnel 104
Captain Nimmo Crepes 105

Vegetables and Side Dishes

Cervical Collard Greens 109
Vertabrussel Sprouts 110
Cervicaliflower and Cheese 111
Whiplashed Potatoes with Pinched Herbes 112
Schmorl's Nodes 113
Praktos Latkes 114
Diversifried Rice 115
Zucchini Foramina Fromagina 116
Spondylitis Onionitis 117
Potatoes o'HIO 118
Nerve Rootabaga 119
Prolapsed Pintos and Peas 120
Toftness Tofu 121
RiSOTto 122
Koren Pudding 123
Achilles Heals 124
Strained Grains and Bowties 125
Crookneck Squash 126
yAKetty yAK yams 127
Websters' Wee Ones 128
Ohm's Baby Carrots with Currants 129
Master's Circle Power Rings 130

Breads

Koren Bread 133
Spoondylitis Bread 134
Snap Crackle Popovers 135
Flexion Bread 136
My Grains Bread 137

Desserts and Sweets

Chocolate Torticollis 141
Sacrumb Cake 142

Scolioatmeal Cookie Logs 143
Energy Cookie Bars 144
Triune Prune Pastry 145
Chocolate Wave Zucchini Bread 146
Chiro Crunch Cookies 147
No Mercy Chocolate Mousse Pie 148
Grassom Grasshopper Pie 149
Big Guy Berry Pie 150
Insurance Bluesberry Cobbler 151
TransMission Fig Nut Bread 152
Sherman Chocolate Cake 153
D. D.'s Double Dipped Mint Cookies 154
Thoracicles 155
Nervana Banana Bread 156
Toggle Toffee 157
Loganberry Crepes 158
Allopathy Taffy 159
National Mixed Fruit Yogurt Pie 160
Gelardi Gelati 161

Straights and Mixers

Sigafoose Juice 165
Centennial Punch 166
Liga Mint Julep 167
Innate Flash 168
Lack of Coordination 169
T4 Two 170
Fountainhead Froth 171
Cloud Walker 172
Fixation 173
Motion Pulpation Spritzers 174
Range of Motion Potion 175
Degeneration 176
Clear View Carrot Juice 177

Glossary 179

Measurements & Substitutions 180

Equivalency Chart 181

Nutrition Basics for a Healthier Life 183

Introduction

This cookbook was first conceived as a vertebral celebration of food and chiropractic. The recipes were created especially for us by a master chef who put scores of hours into developing them. As we ate, innate, innate 'n' ate to sample them, we realized that we had created a nervelle cuisine of spine-tingling recipes to adjust to taste. You'll find that the foods you prepare from these recipes will taste great.

You'll also find that you feel better because humor is a major ingredient in healing. Read more about that in the essay on Humor and Healing. The choices you make will also influence your health, so we've included some useful information on that topic as well.

We hope that these recipes will tickle your funny bone (you'll have to ask your chiropractor where that is!) and that your health will be enhanced.

Cheers!

Beth Coltoff Koren and Tedd Koren, D.C.

Humor and Healing

A happy heart is good medicine and a cheerful mind works healthy, but a broken spirit dries up the bones.—Proverbs 17:22

The arrival of a good clown exercises more beneficial influence upon the health of a town than twenty asses laden with drugs.
—Thomas Sydenham, 17th century physician

People crave laughter as if it were an essential amino acid.
—Patch Adams, MD

Why do we spend millions on prescription drugs each year if our bodies are designed to heal themselves?

It's true. We have a marvelous healing ability that has been shown to heal us of any disease or condition. If we can let it out.

And we can. We have within ourselves incredible means of letting out our inner healing ability. One of the most powerful of these is the universal language: laughter.

Over 25 years ago, Norman Cousins (1915-1990) was diagnosed with a fatal illness. He checked himself out of the hospital and for a fraction of the daily rate checked himself into an expensive hotel, rented a VCR and watched Marx Brothers movies. In his famous book *Anatomy of an Illness*, Cousins described how his pain and disabilities began to recede as laughter washed over his "diseased" body.

"Is it possible," he wondered, "that love, hope, faith, laughter, confidence, and the will to live have therapeutic value?"

Cousins' insights have spawned an industry. The laughter industry. Now scientists are studying the incredible healing effects that a good ol' fashioned happy laugh can do for us.

The more this subject is studied the more profound laughter is found to be.

Laughter, it has been discovered, involves the entire physiology of the body.

Laughter is good for the respiratory system, the cardiovascular system, the muscular system, the central nervous system, the endocrine system, and the immune system.

Laughter makes the brain and body release endorphins, the body's natural painkillers and mood enhancers.

Laughter also can make you healthier. Numerous studies are indicating that a good laugh a day is even better than an apple a day. For example...

In one study people were divided into two groups. One group watched a comedy video; the others sat quietly in a room. Blood samples were drawn every 10 minutes.

The video group had increases in T cells (that battle infection), natural killer cells (that fight infection and cancer), immunoglobulin A antibodies, and gamma interferon immune system chemicals.

The video group also had lower cortisol levels (a stress hormone that suppresses the immune system) and epinephrine (can cause heart palpitations and hypertension).

The non-video group had no changes. [Berk L, Felton D, Tan S et al. Modulators of neuroimmune parameters during the eustress of humor-associated mirthful laughter. *Alternative Therapies.* March 2001;7(2):62-76.]

In addition to fighting disease and improving your resistance laughter exercises your body too. All at the same time?

That's right, in addition to all the changes it makes to your physiology, laughter gives you a good cardio workout, increasing heart activity, lowering blood pressure, and stimulating circulation.

New research even shows that laughter is good for blood sugar levels. No kidding. Diabetics who watched a comedy show had a smaller rise in post-meal blood sugar than when they listened to a non-humorous lecture. The effect occurred in people without diabetes as well. [Hayashi K, Hayashi T, Iwanaga S, Kawai K, Ishii H, Shoji S, Murakami K. Laughter lowered the increase in postprandial blood glucose. *Diabetes Care*. 2003;26(5):1651-1652.]

What an incredible wonder drug! And it's free. Of course you can always see a Broadway show or a Las Vegas revue. Now we're talking money. But I suspect most of our laughter is between friends and loved ones just enjoying everyday life. Maybe that's why life is called "the human comedy."

Why is laughter so good for us? Lots of biological mechanisms are being theorized and a lot of rather dry, decidedly unfunny papers are being published discussing "mirthful laugher" but they'll never get to the heart of the matter.

Why? Because our physiology is only part of the matter of who and what we are. A nice part, but a small part.

The larger part is this:

Laughter, joy, happiness, healing, wholeness, and bliss are our essential nature. It is what we are, our natural state. Did you ever see a bored newborn? Of course not! Babies are closer to their source. They are in touch with the joy, love, bliss, and wonder of being alive.

By expressing those emotions here and now we are connecting to our Source – whatever term you wish to use for that Source. When we laugh we are closer to who we are – an eternal, blissful, immortal being.

Laughter touches our souls and reminds us of who we really are.

breakfasts

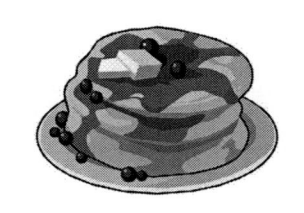

ROMelette with Canadian Bacon

4 large eggs
3 romaine leaves, cut up
¼ lb. Canadian bacon
1 Tbs. butter
salt and pepper to taste

Wash and dry romaine leaves using expansive hand and arm movements. Melt butter in hot pan, add romaine, toss quickly. Beat eggs and add to romaine. Slice or cube bacon and add to mixture. Constantly move mixture in pan until set, fold in half and carefully place on platter. Salt and pepper to taste.

Serves 2.

ROM (range of motion): This range isn't on any ranch. It refers to how far you're able to comfortably move a body part. For example, how far you can turn your head from side to side, up and down, right to left, or sideways. Right to left is your neck (or cervical) range of motion. The same applies to your mid back, low back, hips, even individual vertebrae. All parts that normally move show a range of motion – like arms, legs, fingers and toes. So your jaw has a range of motion, but not your nose. Use your jaw range of motion to enjoy this treat.

Slipped Disc Pancakes with Rotator Cuff Links

1 pkg. link sausages
3 Tbs. flour
¼ tsp. baking powder
⅛ tsp. salt
3 large eggs, separated
5 Tbs. sugar
3 Tbs. milk
1 c. golden delicious apples, cored and diced
1 Tbs. butter
½ tsp. cinnamon

Cook links in skillet according to package directions. Sift together flour, baking powder and salt. Beat egg whites until foamy, not too stiff or dry, then gradually beat in 3 Tbs. sugar until stiff peaks form. Beat egg yolks rotationally until pale and thickened, very slowly add milk. Blend in sifted flour mixture. Fold into egg whites and then fold in apples, gently. Melt butter in large skillet with oven proof handle. Pour in mixture and spread evenly. Sprinkle with remaining sugar and cinnamon. Bake at 375° until set and lightly browned, about 12 minutes. Place on serving platter with the pancakes stacked off center and the sausage links misaligned just so.

Serves 4.

Slipped disc. Discs don't really slip because they're knitted above and below into the vertebrae, so the name slipped disc is really a misnomer. But vertebrae do slip or subluxate and irritate discs.

Discs sorta look like fat pancakes (if you squint a lot) but their fibrous tissue would make them too tough to eat. However it makes a funny breakfast.

Rotator cuff is part of your shoulder joint.

Western States Omelette

3 Tbs. butter
8 large eggs
¼ c. onions, diced
¼ c. green pepper, diced
¼ c. red bell pepper, diced
¼ c. tomatoes, chopped
¼ c. cream
salt and pepper to taste

In a large skillet, melt butter until lightly browned. Beat eggs and stir in remaining ingredients. Pour mixture into hot pan, constantly moving mixture until firm and cooked evenly. Invert onto platter or fold in half and turn out onto platter. Salt and pepper to taste.

Serves 4.

Western States. A chiropractic college in Portland, Oregon. They practice broad spectrum chiropractic there. They also adjust the spine.

Koren Fritters

1 egg, beaten
¼ c. milk
1 c. fresh white corn or 1 c. drained canned corn
1 c. flour
1 tsp. baking powder
½ tsp. salt
½ Tbs. butter or bacon fat, melted
4 slices bacon, cooked crisp and crumbled (optional)
oil for frying

Mix together egg, milk and corn. Add dry ingredients and beat thoroughly. Add butter or fat and blend in bacon. Place 1" of oil in heavy skillet or frying pan. Heat to 375° or hot but not burning. Place heaping tablespoonfuls of mixture into hot oil and fry until golden brown. Drain on paper towels. Serve immediately.

Serves 2 - 4.

Koren. No, it's not Korean, though my family was in dry cleaning years ago. Isn't that the way lots of immigrants made it? They came to America, the promised land, to play handball in Brighton Beach in Brooklyn, press pants, and yell at their kids to go to college and "make something of themselves."

Thomps on Toast

3 large eggs
⅔ c. milk
1 tsp. cinnamon
4 slices bread, at least 1" thick
2 Tbs. butter
1 Tbs. brown sugar
½ c. Thompson grapes
½ c. raisins
½ c. walnuts
2 tbs. maple syrup

Beat together eggs and milk, add cinnamon. Dip slices of bread into mixture and soak for ½ minute on each side. Heat 1 Tbs. butter in medium hot skillet, fry each slice 2 to 3 minutes per side until golden brown. In a saucepan or skillet, melt 1 Tbs. butter, add brown sugar, grapes, raisins and walnuts, toss and heat for 2 to 3 minutes, stir in maple syrup. Place toast on platter and pour fruit/nut mixture over top.

Serves 4.

Clay Thompson, D.C. was one of those multitalented geniuses who made many contributions to chiropractic in many different areas. An associate of B.J. Palmer and the Palmer School of Chiropractic, he developed many adjusting tables and has a technique, the "Thompson Technique."

Mabel Syrup

2 c. maple syrup
1 Tbs. butter
1 cinnamon stick
dash nutmeg
1 tsp. orange zest, chopped or minced

Simmer all ingredients in a saucepan for 5 minutes; stir often. Remove cinnamon stick and serve. Great on waffles, pound cake, sautéed apples, Thomps on Toast (see page 23) or Slipped Disc Pancakes (see page 20).

Makes 2 cups.

Mabel Heath Palmer, D.C. Wife of B.J. Palmer and "founding mother" of chiropractic. Anatomist, author (*Chiropractic Anatomy*, 1918), lecturer, and pioneer women's leader, she had the cool head and temperament needed to translate B.J.'s visions into reality.

hors d'oeuvres & snacks

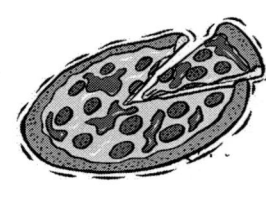

Spine-akopita

1 pkg. filo dough, thawed (keep moist with damp towel on top)
1 c. clarified butter
1 egg, beaten
2 c. feta cheese, crumbled
1 10 oz. pkg. frozen chopped spinach, thawed and drained

Brush cookie sheet with butter. Mix together egg, cheese and spinach. Take one sheet of filo, brush with melted butter, fold in half to make a square. Place one Tbs. of mixture at left corner of dough, fold up corner to make a triangle, fold that half over to right side, then fold up right corner (making another triangle) and fold upwards. Take right corner and fold over to the left. Now you have your triangle! Not as difficult as it sounds once you've done a few. Repeat until mixture is gone. Brush triangles with more butter. Bake at 350° for about 30 minutes, until golden brown.

Makes about 30 triangles.

Spine. Also called the vertebral column, the spinal column or the "backbone." It's made up of 7 neck vertebrae (or spinal bones), 12 thoracic or mid-back vertebrae, 5 lumbars, a sacrum and a coccyx (tailbone). The vertebrae stack up like a pile of donuts with the holes lined up to form a canal, the neural canal, where the spinal cord lies.

Hip Chips

3 large already baked potatoes, day old is best
1 c. vegetable oil
salt and paprika to taste

Heat oil in large skillet. Slice cold potatoes ¼" thick; they will have a star shape in the center. Fry in oil approximately 4 minutes each side until browned and crisp. Drain on paper towels. Sprinkle with salt and paprika. Serve immediately.

Serves 4.

Hip. Your hips are a group of bones surrounding your sacrum (at the base of your spine). You sit on your hips, swing your hips when you dance and need them to hold up your pants. Your legs connect to them – femur head of your thigh goes into the acetabulum of your hip – like a ball and socket. You'd be so lonely without them.

Bone Crackers

whole wheat pita bread
olive oil
garlic powder
oregano, dry and crushed
parmesan cheese (optional)

Cut pita into 1" strips, then carefully separate in half. Place inside up on baking sheet. Drizzle or brush with oil, sprinkle with garlic, oregano, then parmesan cheese. Bake at 350° for about 10 to 12 minutes until crisp. Cool.

Great served with Tedd's Spread (see page 37).

Makes approximately 10 to 12 crackers per pita.

Bone. Those hard things under our skin – where would Halloween be without them?

Crackers? Ugh!, don't call chiropractors "bone crackers." Some respect, please. Calling us that makes us all weepy-eyed.

Lillard Liver Pate

1 lb. chicken livers, washed and patted dry
1 medium onion, chopped
¾ c. chicken stock
2 eggs
¼ c. flour
¼ c. butter, melted
½ c. heavy cream
2 Tbs. cognac
2 tsp. salt
1 tsp. pepper
½ tsp. allspice

Simmer livers and onions in stock for 5 minutes until done. Do not overcook. Add remaining ingredients and pour into a blender. Whirl until smooth, about 1 to 2 minutes, at high speed. Pour mixture into well greased 1 quart loaf pan, cover with foil, and set into pan of hot water making a bain marie. Bake in a slow 325° oven, for 3 hours. Remove and cool. Chill 8 hours or overnight. Slice thin, serve with crisp bread or toast.

Serves 6 - 8.

Harvey Lillard was the first chiropractic patient. He didn't plan on it; it was a supreme act of serendipity. Lillard worked in the building where Dr. D.D. Palmer had his successful magnetic healing office. Lillard experienced a minor accident and had gone deaf 17 years earlier when he felt something give in his back. Palmer found a "bump" in Lillard's spine and adjusted it away. Voila, Lillard's hearing returned. The rest, as they say, is history.

Life Party Mix

1 c. pitted prunes, quartered
1 c. Turkish apricots, quartered
2 c. raisins
1 c. dates, quartered
1 c. pecan pieces
1 c. almonds
1 c. walnut pieces
1 c. sunflower seeds, unsalted
1 c. dried banana chips

Mix all ingredients in extra large bowl. Store in airtight container. Invite everyone you know and open the container.

Makes 10 cups.

Life University in Marietta (near Atlanta) Georgia was the largest of all the chiropractic schools. Their enrollment crashed when they had a mild disagreement with an accrediting agency; now they are on the mend and coming back. They've got a lot to celebrate, which must be why they party so well. The above recipe may be a pre-requisite for enrollment – check your student handbook.

Flesia Pizza

Crust
1 pkg. yeast
3 c. flour (add'l. for kneading)
1½ c. warm water
pinch of salt
oil

Sauce
28 oz. can crushed tomatoes
2 tsp. garlic powder or 3 cloves, crushed
2 tsp. oregano
½ tsp. salt

Topping
8 oz. shredded mozzarella
4 oz. parmesan or locatelli, grated
1 green pepper, sliced
1 onion, sliced thin
½ c. olives, sliced

Crust
In a small bowl, dissolve yeast in warm water. Put flour and salt in a large bowl. Slowly add yeast mixture to flour. Mix by hand, turn onto flour board. When mixture is sticky but holds together add additional flour until dough becomes smooth (about 1½ to 2 cups depending on weather conditions). Knead 8 to 10 minutes. Grease a large bowl with oil, add dough and cover with plastic wrap and a dish towel. Put in a warm place to rise until doubled (about 1½ hours). Punch dough down and let rise again, another 1½ hours. Knead again on floured board until smooth. Cut in half and roll out on floured surface. Oil 2 pizza pans or cookie sheets and place dough round or square on each.

Sauce
In a saucepan, mix ingredients together. Simmer 30 minutes, cool.

Pizza
Place ½ of sauce on each pie. Add cheeses and sliced vegetables. Bake in preheated oven at 450° for 15-20 minutes, until hot and bubbly. Makes 2 pizzas.

Joseph Flesia, D.C., one of the most inspiring speakers in chiropractic, co-created Renaissance International (with Guy Reikeman, D.C.) in the mid '70s which created some of the most ground-breaking chiropractic educational materials the profession has ever seen. A true Renaissance man himself, Dr. Flesia, though he died in 2004, has made a lasting impression on his beloved profession.

Bird Barge

1 large eggplant
3 eggs
½ c. milk
Italian bread crumbs
1½ lb. chicken tenders
oil for frying

Cut eggplant in half lengthwise; scoop out center of one half, leaving a ½" border. Discard center portion. Cut second half of eggplant into finger length and width pieces; trim off skin if you wish. Heat oil in large skillet, about 1" deep. Mix eggs with milk, dip eggplant slices into mixture, then coat with bread crumbs. Fry until crisp. Do the same with the chicken tenders. Keep warm in a 375° oven until all is fried. Place chicken and eggplant in the reserved shell and serve.

Serves 6.

Fred Barge, D.C. was a man of many hats and talents: chiropractor, author, columnist, former President of the International Chiropractors Association, lecturer, researcher and speaker. When Dr. Fred spoke, thousands listened.

spreads, sauces & dips

Tedd's Spread

1 lb. lump crab meat
2-3 Tbs. mayonnaise
1 Tbs. white horseradish
1 tsp. green onion, chopped or sliced thin
1 slice pimento, chopped
dash hot sauce (optional)

Pick over crab meat gently and discard any shells, trying not to break up lumps. Mix together remaining ingredients and gently add crab meat. Chill 1 hour.

Serve with Koren Bread (see page 133).

Serves 8.

Tedd Koren, D.C., is the only Tedd with two ds in the chiropractic profession. Tedd has been widely published in chiropractic journals, philosophically influencing a huge audience. Dr. Koren's interdisciplinary research has been published and read worldwide. He is an international lecturer.

Subloxated Cream Cheese Spread

1 tsp. green onion, chopped
8 oz. cream cheese
¼ c. sour cream
4 oz. lox (nova scotia or smoked salmon)
¼ tsp. dill
black olives, sliced

Mix together green onion, cream cheese, sour cream, lox and dill until smooth. Chill 2 hours. Mold into log or ball and decorate with olive slices.

Serve with Koren Bread (see page 133), crackers, or on top of cucumber rounds.

Makes 1½ cups.

Subluxation. Vertebral subluxation complex, articular joint dysfunction with a neurological component, i.e. bad bone, bad nerve.

Orthodips

8 oz. cream cheese
½ c. mayonnaise
½ c. parsley, chopped
1 egg, hard cooked and cooled, separated
2 Tbs. green onion, sliced thin
1 Tbs. red pepper, chopped (hot or sweet)
1 anchovy, chopped
pepper to taste or 3 drops hot sauce

Beat cream cheese, slowly add mayonnaise, blending well. Add parsley, chopped egg white, green onion, red pepper, anchovy and pepper. Chill 2 hours. Sprinkle with chopped egg yolk.

Makes 2 cups.

Ortho means "straight" or "correct." An orthodontist straightens teeth, an orthopedist straightens bones (like broken ones). Orthopedics is that branch of medicine dealing with structure. They do back and joint surgery, and clash with chiropractors over spinal care. The chiropractors are right. An orthotic is a device that helps keep you straight and balanced. It could be a heel lift, a neck collar or any kind of many different instruments.

Cranialberry Sauce

12 oz. cranberries
½ c. sugar
½ c. water
½ c. orange juice, fresh
2 Tbs. lemon juice, fresh
¾ c. pure maple syrup
⅔ c. dates, pitted and chopped
1 c. pecans, toasted and coarsely chopped

Combine cranberries, sugar, water, orange juice and lemon juice in 8" square baking dish. Stir to blend. Cover tightly and bake in 375° oven until cranberries are very tender, about 40 minutes. Crush most of the cranberries with the back of a spoon. Stir in maple syrup and dates. Bake, uncovered, for 5 minutes. Remove from oven and stir in pecans. Keeps in refrigerator for a couple of weeks.

Serves 6 - 8.

Cranial: pertaining to the head or cranium. Also called your cranial vault because your most prized and valuable possession, your brain, is kept safe and sound there. It is made up of many bones that were once thought to be fused but in reality move a little bit. They can be adjusted using special cranial adjusting techniques.

Manipulated Mangoes

3 mangoes
2 peaches
1 c. orange juice, or other fruit juice
¼ c. peach schnapps

Peel mangoes and peaches. Slice big chunks from the mangoes, getting close to the large pit. Cut peaches in half, remove pit and slice or dice into large pieces. Add fruit juice and schnapps. Heat together in a saucepan 10 minutes on low to medium heat. Do not boil. Cool. Great hot over chicken or pancakes, and hot or cold on ice cream.

Serves 4 - 6.

A **manipulation** is not to be confused with a specific chiropractic spinal adjustment. A spinal adjustment is a very careful realignment of your spine that is preceded by a spinal analysis. A manipulation is just moving something around.

salads

Sid's Caesar

1 large head romaine or 10 oz. bag spinach
1 egg
¼ c. olive oil
1 Tbs. Dijon mustard
1 lemon
1 tsp. Worcestershire sauce
¼ c. parmesan or locatellli, grated
fresh cracked pepper

Wash and dry romaine or spinach. Mix together egg and olive oil, stir in mustard, Worcestershire sauce and the juice of ½ lemon. Pour over greens, toss. Add cheese and cracked pepper. Taste. If you like it a bit more tart, add juice of remaining lemon and toss again.

Serves 4.

Sid Williams, D.C. Irrepressible, charismatic, fearless founder and former President of Life University, the Life Foundation, former president of the International Chiropractors Association and former football player who was called "killer." Who else would name a school "Life?"

Hearts of Palmer Salad

1 large head romaine
1 grapefruit
1 avocado
1 can hearts of palm
½ c. oil
2 Tbs. vinegar
1 tsp. dry mustard
salt and pepper to taste

Wash and dry romaine, tear into bite size pieces. Peel and section grapefruit. Peel and slice avocado. Drain hearts of palm and slice. Mix together oil, vinegar, mustard salt and pepper. Arrange hearts of palm, grapefruit and avocado slices on greens. Pour vinaigrette over salad.

Serves 4.

Palmer. The first family of chiropractic. D.D. Palmer is the "Discoverer" of chiropractic. He was a magnetic healer who constantly looked for new ways to help suffering humanity. His son B.J. was known as the "Developer" of chiropractic, turning it into a force to be reckoned with. Dave Palmer succeeded his father B.J. as head of Palmer College.

Regenerated Sprouts

Salad
2 heads Boston or butterhead lettuce
1 bunch watercress, stemmed
1 avocado, sliced
2 green onions, sliced
1 tsp. chives, chopped
½ c. Roquefort cheese, crumbled
½ c. walnut pieces
2 c. sprouts, home grown is best

Dressing
½ c. sugar
1 tsp. salt
1 c. vegetable oil
1 tsp. dry mustard
1½ Tbs. poppy seeds
⅓ c. apple cider vinegar
½ small onion, minced
1 tsp. honey

Salad
Rinse and pat dry greens. Place in large bowl or on individual plates. Toss with dressing. Top greens with cheese and walnuts. Generously heap sprouts on top and serve with extra dressing.

Dressing
Mix all ingredients and shake until well blended. Makes 2 cups.

Serves 4.

Regeneration: the power to heal. The mystery of life and health is in the science of regeneration. It is one of the cutting edge fields of healthcare and holds the secrets for more than the cure of disease but the restoration of one's health, the reconnection to our Source of life.

Radiculitis Salad

2 heads radicchio, rinsed and patted dry
¼ c. fresh basil leaves
1 endive
6 radishes, thinly sliced
1 onion, thinly sliced
1 Tbs. parsley, chopped
1 pt. cherry tomatoes
1 c. vinaigrette dressing or other
½ c. pitted olives, sliced

Basic vinaigrette
⅔ c. vegetable oil
⅓ c. apple cider vinegar
½ tsp. salt
¼ tsp. fresh cracked pepper
1 clove garlic, crushed

Salad
Arrange radicchio, basil and endive on platter or individual plates. In small bowl toss radishes, onions, parsley and tomatoes with ½ c. of dressing; place on top of lettuce. Sprinkle with olive slices and serve with remainder of dressing.

Dressing
Mix all ingredients. Adjust to suit your taste. Makes 1 cup.

Serves 4.

Radiculitis: inflammation of the root of a spinal nerve. Oooh, that must hurt. And the pain can go all the way around your body, into your arms and legs to your fingers and toes and shoulders and neck. It radiates. Not a fun thing. A cute play on the word radicchio, isn't it?

Lettuce Adjust You Salad

1 head red leaf lettuce
1 head romaine
½ red cabbage
1 cucumber, sliced
1 pt. cherry tomatoes
2 carrots, sliced
10 radishes, sliced
½ cauliflower, cut into florets
1 green bell pepper, julienned
1 midget salami, diced
½ lb. cheddar or other hard cheese, diced
1 can pitted black olives
2 pkgs. Good Seasons cheese and garlic dressing
oil
vinegar

Clean lettuce and pat dry. In extra large bowl, break lettuce into bite size pieces. Add vegetables, meat and cheese. Prepare dressing according to directions. Pour dressing over salad and toss well, but gently. Adjust salad by deleting or adding other vegetables or meats and cheeses to taste. Great to double or triple for a barbecue, luncheon or light supper.

Serves 8 - 10.

Hey, you need an **adjustment**. Lettuce adjust you.

sandwiches

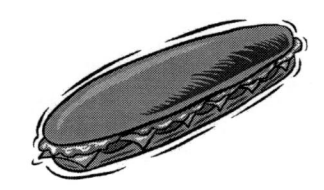

Luxation Sub

2 long Italian rolls
4 oz. cooked salami
4 oz. cooked ham
3 oz. peppered ham
4 oz. provolone or other cheese
shredded lettuce
thinly sliced tomatoes
2 Tbs. oil
1 Tbs. vinegar
1 Tbs. oregano, crushed
⅛ tsp. paprika
sliced hot peppers (optional)

Slice rolls in half lengthwise and scoop out soft inside. Divide meats and cheeses in half. First place meat on roll in layers, then spread out slices of cheese, add lettuce, then tomatoes. Mix together oil, vinegar, oregano and paprika. Sprinkle on top of tomatoes, add hot pepper slices if desired.

Serves 2.

Subluxation, also known as vertebral subluxation complex, spinal nerve stress etc., is a spinal distortion caused when a vertebra loses alignment and irritates, impinges, pinches or interferes with the nerves it was designed to protect. The result is body disharmony: loss of wholeness or dis-ease. Subluxations are caused by stress – a physical accident, poor nutrition, lack of sleep, poor posture, birth stress, emotional upset, etc.

Chronic Club

6 slices whole wheat or rye bread
6 oz. sliced turkey breast
4 oz. smoked ham
4 slices bacon, cooked crisp
2 oz. Swiss cheese
sliced tomatoes and lettuce
2 Tbs. mayonnaise
1 Tbs. mustard
1 tsp. horseradish or dash of hot sauce

Mix mayonnaise, mustard and horseradish or hot sauce together. Start with 2 slices of bread, spread sauce on each piece, divide turkey in half and place slices on bread, then ham. Place another slice of bread on top of each, spread more sauce on each, then use 2 slices of bacon and 1 oz. or slice of cheese on each. Top with tomatoes, lettuce, sauce and 1 slice of bread each. Secure with toothpicks and cut diagonally.

Serves 2.

Chronic: a condition of long-standing duration. It's the opposite of acute which means sudden. The acute desire for this sandwhich was caused by your chronic love of horseradish.

Axis

2 bagels
¼ lb. salami or turkey salami
¼ lb. jarlsberg cheese, sliced
sweet-hot mustard

Slice bagels in half. Spread each half with mustard to taste. Alternately place a slice of cheese, then a slice of salami on each bagel half until all salami and cheese are used. Bake in 300° oven or toaster oven until cheese is melted, approximately 3 to 5 minutes. Remove from oven and put halves together to make sandwiches.

Serves 2.

Axis. The second cervical or neck vertebrae, C-2 or number two under the skull. The axis, true to its name, permits a lot of movement of your head. It was once called the epistropheous (Greek for "the pivot") but is no longer called that in anatomy books.

Knuckle Sandwich

2 Italian rolls
1 Tbs. butter or oil
12 oz. knuckle meat, sliced thin (frozen steak sandwich meat)
salt and pepper to taste
hot pepper, optional
cheese, optional

Slice rolls in half and toast under broiler 1 - 2 minutes. Heat butter or oil in large skillet and sauté just until done, add salt and pepper to taste. Place half of meat in center of each roll, place peppers on top, then cheese of your choice. Place under broiler for 2 minutes until cheese melts.

Serves 2.

Knuckle sandwich, a favorite in NYC. Hey, don't start with me – watch it buster.

The Rondberger or The Peterson Patty

2 Tbs. olive oil
1 med. onion, diced
⅓ lb. mushrooms, chopped
2 tsp. old bay seasoning
1 can pink salmon
2 Tbs. Italian bread crumbs
1 large egg, beaten
3 hamburger rolls

In sauté pan, heat 1 Tbs. oil, add onion and mushrooms, and sauté quickly on medium high light for 4 - 5 minutes. Add old bay seasoning. Cool. In medium bowl, drain and flake salmon, removing any hard bones or skin. Add onion mixture, bread crumbs and egg. Mix well. Form 3 flat patties and cook on medium heat, 4 minutes each side. Place on rolls and serve.

Serves 3.

Terry Rondberg, D.C. is the publisher of *The Chiropractic Journal*. **Donald Peterson** is the editor of *Dynamic Chiropractic*. Both publications are tabloid style newspapers that are often on opposite sides of the chiropractic political spectrum.

The American Chiropractor Hot Dog

4 thick slices bacon or beef fry
1 onion, thinly sliced
4 kosher knockwurst hot dogs
4 slices American cheese
1 Tbs. mustard
1 Tbs. ketchup
4 short hoagie rolls

Cook bacon in fry pan on low heat just until opaque – do not crisp. Remove bacon and set aside. In same pan, add onions to bacon drippings, sauté on medium low heat until soft, about 2 - 3 minutes. Remove onions and keep warm.

Make a slit in each hot dog (avoid cutting through bottom and edges). Cut slices of cheese in half, lay end to end and place inside hot dog. Wrap 1 slice of half cooked bacon around each hot dog, secure with toothpick, keeping cheese covered with bacon. Fry in pan until bacon is cooked completely and is crisp, about 6 minutes. Combine mustard and ketchup, spread on rolls. Place hot dog in roll and top with your choice of condiments. Serve immediately.

Serves 4.

The American Chiropractor magazine is one of the popular publications of the chiropractic profession.

soups & stews

Lumbar Jack Soup

1 c. dried pea or pinto beans
2 qts. water
¼ c. oil
1 c. celery, diced
1 c. carrots, diced
1 c. onions, diced
26 oz. can tomatoes
1 can corn
1 clove garlic, minced
⅓ c. parsley, chopped
2 tsp. salt
¼ tsp. pepper
½ c. ditalini pasta

Wash beans and pick over, drain. Cover beans with 2 quarts of water, bring to a boil for 2 minutes. Heat oil in large kettle. Add celery, carrots, onions, corn, tomatoes and garlic. Sauté lightly. Add beans, water and remaining ingredients. Cook covered for 2½ to 3 hours. Makes about 2½ quarts.

Serves 6 - 8.

Lumbar. Your low back vertebrae, located between your sacrum and thoracic spine. They're big, they're strong and they're mean (especially when they subluxate). They carry a lot of weight. Be nice to them. Honor them by eating the above soup.

Gonstead Gumbo

1 4 lb. chicken, cut into 8-10 pieces
1 Tbs. salt
1 tsp. pepper
1 clove garlic, smashed
4 oz. salt pork
1 red bell pepper, diced
1 c. onion, diced
¼ c. flour
2⅓ c. can tomatoes (19 oz. can)
1 10 oz. package frozen okra or 1 can, drained
1 lb. raw shrimp, cleaned
hot sauce

Cook chicken in 6 cups water with salt, pepper and garlic for 2½ to 3 hours, until tender. Cool. Debone meat and cut into chunks. Keep broth and add more water to make 6 cups, cool and skim off fat. Heat salt pork until browned. Remove pork and set aside. Sauté red pepper and onion in large frying pan with lid for 5 minutes. Add flour, toss and brown. Slowly stir in broth, tomatoes and pork. Cover and simmer for 30 minutes. Add chicken chunks, okra and shrimp. Simmer, covered, for approximately 5 minutes until shrimp are pink. Season to taste with hot sauce.

Serve over rice.

Serves 4.

Clarence Gonstead, D.C. A big man who developed the Gonstead technique. To a little village where he practised in Mt. Horeb, Wisconsin people from around the world came to benefit from his miraculous adjusting technique while doctors traveled far and wide to sit at his feet. His was one of the most successful clinics in the profession – he had to build an airport and a hotel to accommodate the crowds.

Lambago Stew

2 lbs. lamb shoulder
⅔ c. flour
½ tsp. salt
¼ tsp. pepper
2 Tbs. vegetable oil
¾ c. onion, diced
5 tomatoes, cubed
2 bay leaves
2 Tbs. barley
1 clove garlic
1 tsp. paprika
1 c. water or beef broth

Trim fat off meat and cube. Mix flour with salt and pepper, dredge meat lightly. Heat oil in kettle. Add onions, cook until tender, not brown, then add meat and remaining ingredients. Cover and simmer for 2 hours adding water or broth a little at a time if it begins to dry out. Continue cooking until meat is tender.

Serves 4.

Lumbago is an old term for lower back aches. Sometimes you'll hear an actor in an old movie talk about his lumbago. "Mah lumbago's a mite testy tonight, momma." As a kid I thought he was referring to an old car he owned.

Cartilegume Soup

2 c. split peas
2 onions, chopped
6 c. water
3 c. chicken stock
½ c. crushed peanuts
salt and pepper to taste
curry powder

Wash peas and pick over. Boil peas and onions in water for 30 minutes. Simmer 1½ hours. Puree and return to pot. Add stock, season to taste. Top with crushed peanuts and sprinkle with curry powder.

Serves 4 - 6.

Cartilage. Cute turn of a phrase, huh? Cartilage is that stuff that sits on joints that's used to make glue and jello. Now you know why they sold your pony.

Parker 'n' Beans

1 lb. dried lima beans
6 c. water
¾ lb. bacon, diced
1 onion, diced
1 green pepper, diced
1 green onion, diced
1 Tbs. flour
1 tsp. salt
¼ tsp. pepper
2 tsp. yellow mustard
1 tsp. Worcestershire sauce
2-3 Tbs. brown sugar (to taste)
2⅓ c. tomatoes (19 oz. can)

Wash beans, pick over. Cover beans with 6 cups water, bring to a boil for 2 minutes. Remove from heat, cover for 1 hour, then cook again until tender. Drain. Cook bacon until crisp. Remove and save. Add onions and pepper to bacon fat, cook 4 - 5 minutes. Add flour, salt, pepper, mustard and Worcestershire, stir well. Add tomatoes and simmer for 15 minutes. Add beans, cook another 10 - 15 minutes. Top with crispy bacon.

Serves 6.

It's stupendous! It's colossal! It's **Parker!** Who else can get thousands of chiropractors, wives and C.A.'s under one roof at one time? It's a twenty-ring show. And it all started as a small get together of brown-bagging doctors.

B.J.'s X-ray Consommé

1 roaster chicken
2 celery ribs with leaves
2 carrots
sprig of dill
1 parsnip
1 turnip
2 medium onions
salt and pepper to taste

Cut chicken into 11 pieces including the back and neck. Clean chicken parts thoroughly. Place in large pot and cover with water. Cut up vegetables and lay on top of chicken (with enough water to keep covered), bring to a gentle boil, then simmer for 2 hours. Discard vegetables and remove chicken. De-bone meat and put bones back into pot, simmer for at least one more hour, add salt and pepper to taste. Strain soup and refrigerate overnight. Skim off all fat, return to a pot and heat. Adjust seasoning, strain again to achieve a clear broth. Leftover chicken makes excellent chicken salad.

Makes approximately 1½ quarts.

B. J. Palmer, son of D.D. Palmer, (the Discoverer of Chiropractic) has been described as part showman, part scientist and all chiropractor. He, more than any single person, saved chiropractic from medical annihilation. He said, "I will serve chiropractic, save chiropractic if it will take me twenty lifetimes to do it." He packed all his lifetimes in one incredible career. His work has had a powerful influence on every aspect of chiropractic philosophy, science and art. Love him or hate him, you couldn't ignore him.

X-ray (sorta rhymes with consommé): a way of seeing through people. How do you do it? Easy. Stick someone in front of an x-ray tube, press the button and zap, on the other side is an exposed film of....shadows. Well, that's what an x-ray is, a lot of shadows. But what shadows!

Quack Soup

1 duck, 4½ to 5 lbs., cut up and reserve breast meat
2 carrots, cut in 1" dice
1 onion, quartered
1 celery stalk w/leaves, cut in 1" dice
water
1 tsp. salt
½ tsp. pepper

1 qt. chicken stock
4 oz. cepes or other dried mushrooms
2 Tbs. Madeira
2 Tbs. hot water
3 Tbs. clarified butter
2 Tbs. flour
1 c. cream

Place duck parts (except breast) with carrots, onion and celery in a large stock pot and cover with water. Add salt and pepper, bring to a boil and simmer for 2 hours. Remove meat (save for a cold duck salad) and vegetables. Strain broth and chill. Skim off all fat and discard. Add chicken stock to duck broth and simmer another hour to reduce; taste and season accordingly. Meanwhile, soak mushrooms in Madeira and hot water for ½ hour. Remove mushrooms; save liquid. Rinse and drain them; chop. In very hot pan, sauté breasts approximately 10 minutes per side until cooked slightly pink inside. Remove skin and slice thin. Keep warm. Place butter and flour in sauté pan, stirring (to make a roux) until incorporated. Slowly add reserved mushroom liquid, simmer and add cream, stirring to keep smooth. Add reduced stock and simmer 5 minutes. Adjust seasoning if needed. Place soup in serving bowls, top with sliced duck pieces and mushrooms. Serve hot.

Serves 6.

Hey, you gotta be able to laugh at yourself. So I don't want any nasty letters. Actually a **quack** is someone who pretends to medical expertise. Chiropractors make no such pretense; they are experts in chiropractic. Hence they cannot be quacks. See? I told you so.

The word quack is from quacksalver or quicksilver – also known as mercury. It was applied to dentists who used mercury amalgam as opposed to those who used gold and silver. They were considered quacks for putting a poisonous substance into people's mouths.

Koren Chowder

3 c. good chicken stock
3 c. fresh corn
¼ c. butter
¼ c. onion, diced
1 clove garlic, crushed
1 tsp. sugar
1 c. potatoes, diced and cooked
2 c. light cream
1 tsp. dill
salt and pepper

In large saucepan or pot, simmer chicken stock. Scrape kernels from corn and add to stock; cover and continue simmering for 5 minutes. Heat butter in sauté pan with onion and garlic for 5 minutes until opaque and softened. Add sugar and stir mixture into stock. Simmer 15 more minutes. Add potatoes, cream and dill. Season with salt and pepper.

Serves 6.

What can you say about **Tedd Koren** that he hasn't said about himself already? An explorer, a rock star, a movie actor, an archeologist, a talented baseball player – they all live in his neighborhood.

cheeses & pastas

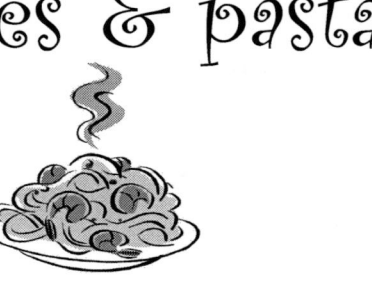

Pasta Verdebra

1 lb. green (spinach) linguine
6 oz. butter
2 green onions, chopped
½ c. parsley, chopped
pepper to taste

Cook pasta according to directions, drain. Heat butter, add green onion, parsley and pasta. Toss and serve immediately.

Serves 4 - 6.

Vertebra. Your back bones. They make up your spine and look a little like signet rings (if you squint real hard). Dem bones gon rise. I think that's from an old spiritual. Oh well.

Gouda-justment Soufflé

4 large eggs, plus 1 egg white
1¼ c. gouda cheese, finely grated
salt and pepper
3 Tbs. butter plus enough to coat soufflé dish
3 Tbs. flour
½ tsp. dry mustard
1 c. milk

Separate eggs and leave at room temperature, covered, for 1 hour. Preheat oven to 375°. Butter a 6 cup soufflé dish and coat with ¼ c. grated cheese. Set aside. Melt 3 Tbs. butter, add flour (to make a roux), stir constantly and cook 2 minutes until well blended. Add mustard and milk, stir until thick and smooth. Remove from heat. With a wire whisk, vigorously beat in 1 egg yolk at a time, then add remaining cup of cheese. Put on low heat, stir 2 minutes. Leave at room temperature. Beat egg whites (in a copper bowl if possible) until light and airy, shiny and stiff-peaked but not dry. Add ¼ of the egg whites to cheese mixture, blend carefully but completely to lighten batter. Fold in remainder of egg whites. Quickly place mixture into soufflé dish. Run finger around rim to make an indentation or collar. Place in middle of oven on lowest rack. Bake 25 to 30 minutes, until almost firm in center, or firmer if you prefer. Serve immediately.

Serves 2 as an entree, 4 as a side dish.

And may all your **adjustments** be gouda.

Spiney Lobster and Linguine

8 rock lobster tails (spiny lobster), 4-5 oz. each
water
salt
½ c. butter
1 c. cream
¼ c. onion, chopped
1 clove garlic, chopped
1 Tbs. parsley, chopped
¼ tsp. pepper
1 lb. linguine

Prepare linguine according to directions, rinse and drain. Set aside. Boil lobster in salted water for 10 minutes, until firm and pink. Drain. Cut shell, remove meat and slice into medallions or chunks. Melt butter with cream, add onion, garlic, parsley and pepper. Stir in lobster meat, heat 2 minutes. Add linguine, toss and serve immediately.

Serves 4 - 6.

Spine. When the ancient geeks, er, Greeks, looked at peoples' backs they saw a lot of bumps that reminded them of thorns (spina in Greek — see also Spine-akopita, page 27). I've often wondered where those Greeks got their ideas, I mean, the constellations don't look anything like bears and dogs and hunters, even if you do connect the dots. What imaginations those Greeks had. See what you can do when you don't have cable to distract you? Incidentally, chiropractors don't have an animal mascot. My vote is for the Spiney Lobster. Or at least this recipe.

Ruptured Rigatoni

1 lb. rigatoni
2 Tbs. olive oil
1 medium onion, chopped
1 green pepper, diced
1 red bell pepper, diced
1 clove garlic, chopped
1 lb. ground chuck or turkey
1 tsp. oregano, crushed
½ tsp. hot red peppers, crushed (more if desired)
1 medium tomato, chopped
2 c. tomato sauce
⅔ c. parmesan cheese, grated

Cook rigatoni, drain and run under cold water to stop cooking. Drain again and set aside in large casserole or baking dish. Heat oil and sauté onion, peppers and garlic until tender but firm. Mix with pasta. In skillet, cook meat. Add oregano, crushed peppers, tomatoes and tomato sauce. Heat mixture 5 minutes. Pour over rigatoni and blend well. Sprinkle with cheese. Bake at 350° covered with foil for 45 minutes. Uncover, bake 15 minutes longer or until browned and bubbly.

Serves 6 - 8.

Rupture. Ugh! Not a good thing. Your disc's way of telling you to find an industrial-strength chiropractor. But this recipe is kidding you. The rigatoni remains intact.

Curves and Whey

1 lb. fusilli
3 Tbs. butter
1 large onion, diced
1 large green pepper, diced
1 c. mushrooms, chopped
1 c. water
1 26 oz. can tomatoes
1 12 oz. can tomato paste
1 tsp. salt
½ tsp. pepper
1½ lb. cheddar cheese, shredded
3 Tbs. parmesan cheese, grated

Cook fusilli according to package directions, drain. Put into 4 quart casserole dish. Sauté onion, green pepper and mushrooms for 10 minutes. Add 1 cup water, tomatoes, tomato paste, salt and pepper. Bring to a boil, pour over fusilli. Stir and add cheddar cheese. Stir again then sprinkle parmesan on top. Bake at 350° for 1½ hours or until browned and bubbly.

Serves 6 - 8.

When you look at someone from the front or the back their spine should look relatively straight. It's much easier to see if they don't have any clothes or skin or muscles or guts on, that's why X-rays are so popular. But when you look at a person from the side they should have **curves** in their spine – it makes it stronger and more flexible. You normally have three spinal curves, the cervical or lordotic curve in your neck, the thoracic or kyphotic curve in your midback and another lordotic curve in your lower back. Your neck and lower back curve the same way, or they should.

Spinal Spiral Pasta and Peppers

1 lb. spiral pasta (rotelle)
⅓ c. vegetable or olive oil
1 red bell pepper, sliced
1 green pepper, sliced
1 yellow bell pepper, sliced
1 clove garlic, chopped
½ tsp. basil, crushed
salt and pepper to taste
parmesan cheese (optional)

Cook pasta according to package directions, drain. Heat oil in skillet, add pepper slices, garlic and basil. Sauté approximately 6 minutes until tender but still crisp. Add salt and pepper to taste. Pour over pasta and sprinkle with cheese if desired.

Serves 4 - 6.

Spinal: pertaining to the spine, of course. If your spine is spiral shaped you've got one hell of a problem.

Tennis Elbows

8 large plum tomatoes
1 tsp. dried basil
½ tsp. sugar
¼ tsp. salt
1 Tbs. olive oil
8 oz. macaroni
1 Tbs. fresh basil, chopped
2 oz. parmesan or locatelli cheese, in chunk

Preheat oven to 200°. Halve tomatoes lengthwise and place on cookie sheet, cut side up. Mix dried basil, sugar and salt. Sprinkle mixture on top of tomatoes. Bake for 6 - 7 hours. Do not completely dry out.

Prepare macaroni according to package directions. Drain and rinse. Toss with oil and fresh basil. Cut tomatoes in quarters, add to macaroni and toss. Place on serving platter. Grate cheese on top and serve. For a browner, crispier dish, place under broiler for 1 - 2 minutes and serve.

Serves 4.

Elbow: It's not the spine but, hey, your elbow's a joint. What more can we say? It tastes real good (the recipe that is; I don't know about your elbows but mine tend to dry out a little in the winter). Maybe one day we'll have a vertebra shaped macaroni?

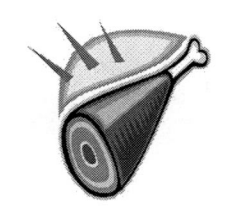

meats

Van Rumpt Roast

3 lb. rump, cut into large cubes, remove fat
1 tsp. salt
¼ c. red wine
1½ c. tomatoes, canned or fresh
1 large onion, quartered
10 small red or white potatoes, peeled
2 cloves garlic
pepper to taste

Put meat and salt into a pot, add red wine, cover. Roast in a preheated 350° oven for 1¾ hours. Add vegetables and garlic. Cover, continue cooking for 1 hour or until all ingredients are tender. Pepper to taste.

Serves 8.

Richard Van Rumpt, D.C. was the developer of the chiropractic analysis and adjusting technique called DNFT, Directional-Non-Force-Technic or simply Van Rumpt. He was a brilliant, feisty old codger who knew his stuff. Van Rumpt's work has influenced many technique researchers.

Misaligned Meatloaf

2 large potatoes, sliced
1 onion, sliced
1 tsp. salt
1½ lbs. ground chuck or turkey
¾ c. bread crumbs
1 c. tomato sauce
2 Tbs. parsley, chopped
1 Tbs. water
1 Tbs. Worcestershire sauce
1 tsp. Dijon mustard
1 Tbs. dry minced onion
1 tsp. garlic powder

Layer potatoes and onions in a 2 quart baking dish, sprinkle with salt. Mix remaining ingredients and spread into pan. Bake, uncovered, at 350° for 1¼ hours.

Serves 4.

Misaligned: out of proper alignment. Some meatheads just can't keep anything straight. A misaligned meatloaf should sell at half-price. But our serious recipe writer just gives you the bare bones. If you want to twist it up for a proper presentation, be our guest.

Short Leg of Lamb

1 4 - 5 lb. leg of lamb, rinsed and dried
8 cloves garlic
8 prunes, pitted
1 Tbs. ginger, grated
½ c. orange juice
salt and pepper

Cut 8 slits in leg of lamb. Stuff each slit with 1 garlic clove and 1 prune. Rub lamb well with salt and pepper. Put on rack in shallow roasting pan. Mix ginger and orange juice together and baste meat every ½ hour or hour. Roast uncovered in preheated 300° oven, 25 minutes per pound for rare, 30 minutes per pound for medium. Rest meat for 20 minutes before slicing and pour over any leftover juices.

Serves 4 - 6.

Short leg. Wanna start a fight? Get a dozen D.C.s from different technique schools together and ask them what the short leg means. Then get under a table or hide behind the bar. After the smoke clears they'll still be fighting. Smile when you ask that question, pardner.

Carver's Delight

2½ lb. center cut filet mignon (boneless)
½ c. butter
1 clove garlic, diced or smashed
2 shallots, diced
1 tsp. salt
¼ tsp. pepper
1 tsp. rosemary

If possible, take sinew off filet and place in shallow roasting pan. Heat butter with remaining ingredients, just until melted. Pour ½ of sauce over filet and roast at 350° for approximately 1 hour or until meat thermometer registers desired doneness. Rest meat for 15 minutes and slice. Pour off any pan drippings into remaining butter sauce, heat for 2 minutes and pour over sliced beef.

Serves 6.

Willard Carver, Esq., D.D. Palmer's lawyer, defended him from jealous M.D.s who didn't like competition. He was so inspired by this new form of healthcare that he became a D.C. himself and went on to develop his own school of spinal analysis and his own schools of chiropractic. Like D.D. he also fought with B.J. Palmer. Ah, tradition.

Tender Ribs

3 lbs. pork ribs, country style
1 Tbs. vegetable oil
1 small onion, diced
1 c. ketchup
½ c. water
2 Tbs. brown sugar
3 Tbs. lemon juice
1 Tbs. Worcestershire sauce
1 Tbs. honey
1 Tbs. cider vinegar
1 clove garlic, crushed
1 tsp. ginger, grated

Cut ribs into single servings, set aside. Heat oil and sauté onion. Add rest of ingredients and simmer 30 minutes. Cool. Pour marinade over ribs and refrigerate for 2 to 3 hours. Bake in preheated 325° oven for 1½ to 2 hours or until tender, then broil or grill for 5 minutes until browned.

Serves 4 - 6.

Ribs. They connect to the 12 thoracic vertebrae of your spine. There are a dozen pairs, 24, in both men and women. No, women don't have one less. I don't know why they say that in the Bible. And I don't care. And I don't want to get any nasty letters.

Ribley Riblets

4 lbs. beef short ribs, separated
⅔ c. flour
1 tsp. salt
½ tsp. pepper
½ tsp. paprika
½ tsp. garlic powder
2 Tbs. oil
1 c. water
½ c. red wine
1 c. carrots. diced
½ c. celery, diced
¼ c. parsley, chopped
1 bay leaf, crushed

Wash and pat dry ribs. Mix flour with salt, pepper, paprika and garlic powder. Dredge (coat lightly) ribs with flour mixture. Heat oil in 5 qt. dutch oven and brown meat on all sides. Add water and wine; add rest of ingredients. Bake covered at 300° for 3 hours or until fork tender. Stir 2 - 3 times while cooking.

Serves 4.

Chuck Ribley, D.C. "River Chuck" is chiropractic's 60's hippy. He was once a straight-laced D.C. but started talking new age stuff and takes people out to the desert and does firewalking and all kinds of things you read about in the *Wall Street Journal*. Hey, far from me to question him – every time I see him he looks pretty happy. Maybe that stuff works?

The Nerve of Ewe

1½ lbs. lamb shoulder
½ c. flour
1 tsp. salt
½ tsp. pepper
½ tsp. garlic powder
½ tsp. paprika
2 Tbs. butter or oil
1 large onion, chopped
1 16 oz. can whole tomatoes
¾ c. water

Rinse lamb, cut into 1" cubes and pat dry. Mix flour with dry spices. Dredge (coat lightly) meat in flour. Melt butter or oil in large saucepan; add lamb and cook over medium heat, browning on all sides for about 8 minutes. Add onions and cook until they are soft and translucent, another 5 - 8 minutes. Add tomatoes, with juice, and water. Reduce heat and simmer about 1½ hours until meat is fork tender. Add more salt and pepper if needed. Stir occasionally. Great over noodles or rice.

Serves 4.

Another one of our witty play on words. **Nerves** are very sensitive cells that transmit electrical-like messages all over your body. There are billions of them in your brain, in fact, they are your brain and their fibers extend outside your skull as a thick cord – the spinal cord. Within them are the secrets of life, death and taxes. Forget about Star Trek, nerves are the final frontier.

Massaged Flank Steak

1 - 2 lb. flank steak
¼ c. light soy sauce
2 Tbs. water or vermouth
1 Tbs. fresh ginger, grated or minced
1 Tbs. fresh garlic, grated or minced
1 ziploc plastic bag

Rinse flank steak and pat dry. Mix soy sauce, water or vermouth, ginger and garlic in plastic bag. Place meat in bag and seal. Massage meat in marinade on both sides and refrigerate for 2 hours. If meat marinates too long it will break down and become mushy. Remove meat and place on broiler pan. Broil as close to flame as possible. Keep door ajar when broiling, to prevent fire or smoking. Turn over after 6 minutes for 4 more minutes or until medium rare. Let rest 2 minutes; slice on the diagonal, against the grain.

Serves 4 - 6.

Massage. It feels great. Gets that old blood moving, drains those tissues of schmutz (toxins), it's even good for the brain. Better than an apple a day for keeping you-know-who away.

poultry

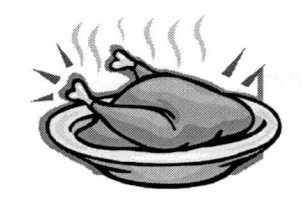

Duck á lo'range of Motion

1 4 - 5 lb. duck
salt, pepper and garlic powder
½ c. orange juice
¼ c. honey
1 orange
parsley

With a meat fork, pierce duck several times, allowing fat to drip out of skin. Rub duck with seasonings. Roast on rack in shallow pan at 325° for 2 hours. Mix orange juice and honey together and baste duck. Raise temperature to 350° and roast for 1 more hour. If fat is splattering, add some water to roasting pan. Peel and slice orange. Halve or quarter duck and serve with orange slices and parsley.

Serves 2.

Range of motion. Hey, we discussed this. Look under omelettes. OK, I'll say something else about it. Hmm…maybe I won't.

Chicken Hips

1 c. plain yogurt
1 Tbs. jalapeno chili (seeded and minced)
1 tsp. ground cumin
¼ tsp. cayenne pepper
6 whole chicken legs (with thighs)

Combine yogurt, jalapeno, cumin and pepper. Wash chicken and pat dry. Coat chicken with yogurt sauce and marinate for 3-4 hours. Bake at 350° for 45 minutes or grill for 30 minutes (until juices run clear) turning at least once. Great with basmati rice.

Serves 4 - 6.

Hips. We discussed that too. I've known chiropractors who adjust all kinds of animals, chickens included.

Bruised Celery Ribs with Chicken

1 4 - 5 lb. chicken, cut into 8 pieces
1 whole stalk celery
1 c. chicken stock
½ Tbs. butter, melted
½ tsp. garlic powder
¼ tsp. salt
⅛ tsp. pepper
½ c. cream
2 Tbs. parsley, chopped
½ tsp. paprika

Rinse chicken pieces and pat dry. Remove tough outer ribs of celery and cut off bottom. Arrange celery in bottom of dutch oven. Add chicken stock, butter, garlic, salt and pepper. Place chicken pieces on top of celery. Bring to a boil, cover and braise (simmer) for 45 - 50 minutes. During cooking baste chicken a few times with cooking juices. Remove chicken. Skin pieces if you wish. Place celery on serving platter; arrange chicken on top or around sides. Bring broth to a boil; add cream and parsley. Stir 1 minute and pour over chicken. Sprinkle with paprika and serve.

Serves 4.

Bruised ribs. Hey, be gentle when you do that adjustment. And watch out if you're playing tackle football.

Knee Jerk Chili

2 - 3 tbs. oil
2 lbs. ground turkey
1 medium onion, diced
1 clove garlic, minced
1 1 lb. can tomatoes
1 6 oz. can tomato paste
2 tsp. chili powder
1 tsp. paprika
¼ tsp. crushed red pepper
2 1 lb. cans red kidney beans
salt and pepper to taste

In a large pot, heat oil, add onion and garlic. Cook 5 minutes, add turkey and cook 15 minutes, stirring often. Add tomatoes, tomato paste, chili powder, paprika and red pepper; stir for 2 minutes. Add beans, cover and simmer 1½ hours. Taste, add salt and pepper as needed.

Serves 6.

Knee jerk. A reflex. That means stuff that goes on in your nerves without your having to think of it. Remember when you pulled your hand away from that hot skillet before you knew it was hot? Reflexes can be pretty fast. Reflexes were once thought to be pretty simple things but spinal cord reflexes are one of the ways an unhealthy spine causes internal organ malfunction, muscle unbalances and general yuckiness. May all your reflexes be happy ones.

Chicken Fingers with Arthrices Stuffing

Stuffing

1 c. cooked brown rice
½ c. cooked wild rice
1 c. bread cubes
3 oz. water chestnuts, drained and chopped
¼ c. chicken stock

1 Tbs. butter
1 small onion, diced
1 celery rib, sliced
1 clove garlic, crushed
½ tsp. dried thyme
salt and pepper to taste

Mix together cooked rices, bread, water chestnuts and stock in large bowl. Heat butter in medium sauté pan, add onion, celery and garlic. Cook on medium heat until transparent, add thyme. Add onion mixture to rice, taste for seasoning and add salt and pepper as needed. Bake covered at 350° for 40 minutes, uncover (if it looks too dry, add a little bit more stock) and bake 10 - 15 minutes longer. Also great for use in a turkey or whole chicken.

Chicken Fingers

1 c. flour
1 tsp. salt
¼ tsp. pepper
1 Tbs. butter, melted
1 egg yolk
10 oz. stale beer

2 egg whites, stiffly beaten
1¼ -1½ lb. chicken tenders
4 drops hot sauce
¼ tsp. cayenne
½ - ¾ c. water
oil for frying

Mix together flour, salt, pepper, butter, egg yolk and beer, beat until smooth. Let rest for 1 - 3 hours. Fold in egg whites just before using. Meanwhile, make marinade for tenders.

Mix together hot sauce, cayenne and water. Dip chicken and marinate at least 1 hour. When ready, remove tenders, pat dry and dip in batter to coat evenly. Heat oil until medium hot but not smoking. Place tenders gradually into hot oil and fry for 5 - 7 minutes. Serves 4.

Osteoarthritis is considered a disease of old age – but that's really not so. If it really were due to age, a person's entire spine would be arthritic, not just a few select areas. It's really due to wear and tear of an unbalanced spine. Don't let that happen to you. Get an adjustment already.

fish & seafood

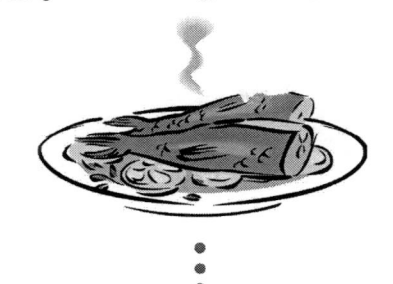

Dorsal Morsels

4 baby salmon or trout, 1 lb. each
½ c. flour
salt, pepper, garlic powder and paprika
½ c. vegetable oil
4 Tbs. butter
2 tsp. garlic, minced
½ c. white wine
2 tsp. parsley, chopped

Make sure fish is clean and dry. Mix flour with seasonings and lightly flour fish. Heat oil and pan-fry fish for 5 minutes, then turn. In a separate pot, heat butter until lightly browned. Add garlic, wine and parsley. Pour over fish and cook 5 more minutes.

Serves 4.

Dorsal. An old term for the mid-back vertebrae. The word thoracic is used more often nowadays to describe the 12 vertebrae that connect to your ribs. Sharks have dorsal fins (that's the fin that sticks out of the water). Perhaps we should call them lawyer fins?

Sacral Mackerel

4 mackerel, ¾ lb. each
½ tsp. salt
½ tsp. dry mustard
¼ tsp. pepper
¼ c. oil
3 Tbs. soy sauce
1 Tbs. ginger, grated or diced

Wash and dry fish, sprinkle inside and out with dry seasonings. Heat oil and pan-fry fish for 5 minutes each side. Mix soy sauce with ginger and pour over fish. Gently sauté for 2 more minutes.

Serves 4.

Sacral, pertaining to the sacrum. The sacrum is in the lower part of your spine. It's made up of five fused vertebrae. Ancient peoples used it to foretell the future, they thought it was a sacred bone. Hence the name.

Pulled Mussels

24 mussels, live and fresh
cold water
2 cloves garlic, smashed
1 19 oz. can tomatoes
2 Tbs. parsley, chopped
¼ c. red wine (optional)

Scrub mussels, debeard and rinse several times in cold water to remove sand and drain. In large pot, heat remaining ingredients for 2 minutes and add mussels. Cook for 10 minutes, until mussels open. Discard any that do not open.

Serve hot over pasta.

Serves 2.

Muscles. Muscles don't push, they only pull. A pulled muscle is really a lay term for a muscle that's pulled a little too much. It's more accurately called a strained muscle.

Loxyx Coccyx

2 lb. raw salmon filet
½ c. fresh lime or lemon juice
1 onion, minced
1 bunch fresh dill
½ c. parsley, chopped
½ tsp. salt
¼ tsp. sugar
¼ c. cider vinegar

Wash filet, pat dry. Place fish in casserole dish, add lime juice and coat completely. Chill 8 hours or overnight in refrigerator. Drain well. Mix remaining ingredients and spread over entire fish. Chill for 4 to 6 hours. Slice very thin.

Serve with buttered pumpernickel.

Serves 8.

Coccyx: what's left of our tailbone. It's made up of a few fused, tiny vertebrae. Sometimes the coccyx extends outside the body as a real human tail. But that's very rare. An old joke: Did you hear about the baby born with a tail? It took the doctors three hours to remove it. The first two were spent getting it down from the chandelier. OK, I never said it was a good joke. But seriously folks.... The coccyx is no vestigial organ but vital for your life and health. For example, the meninges, the coverings of the brain and spinal cord, anchor to the coccyx. Problems with the coccyx could cause problems with your brain. Both ends really are connected.

Gillet Fillets

2 lbs. flounder or other white fish
juice of ½ lemon
¼ c. white wine
½ c. water
salt and pepper to taste
3 Tbs. butter
3 Tbs. flour
1 c. stock
½ c. heavy cream
3 Tbs. gruyere, grated
3 Tbs. locatelli or romano, grated

Sprinkle fillets with lemon juice, salt and pepper, and pour on wine. Add water. Bring to a simmer, covered, and poach for 10 minutes. Pour off liquid and save. Make liquid equal 1 cup by adding water if necessary. Make a roux by melting butter and adding flour, cooking until smooth. Remove from heat and add hot stock. Whisk until smooth again. Add cream, cook until thickened. Pour over fish. Sprinkle cheeses on top and broil until brown, about 3 - 4 minutes.

Serves 4.

Henri Gillet, D.C. of Belgium had a problem. Chiropractors weren't permitted to use x-rays so how to accurately figure out what was going on in the spine? The answer – discover and develop motion palpation. It is now a popular spinal analysis technique.

Carp á la Tunnel

3 Tbs. butter
1 clove garlic, chopped
1 large onion, diced
½ c. mushrooms, diced
½ c. parsley, minced
1 Tbs. bread crumbs
salt and pepper to taste
4 carp fillets, ½ lb. each
1 c. white wine
1 large tomato, diced
1 Tbs. parsley, chopped

Heat butter, add garlic, onion and mushrooms. Sauté 3 to 4 minutes and add bread crumbs, parsley salt and pepper. Sauté 2 more minutes. Wash and dry each fillet. Place ¼ of stuffing mixture onto each fillet and roll up. Heat white wine with tomato and parsley in pan, place rolled fillets on top and simmer 8 to 10 minutes until firm but flaky.

Serves 4.

Carpal tunnel. You won't find this tunnel on a road map. It's created by the bones of the wrist. Pretty good play on words, huh? Carpal Tunnel Syndrome, also known as repetitive stress disorder, is an often painful condition of the wrist where nerves in the wrist are trapped in the wrist or carpal tunnel. Interestingly, a cervical (neck) spinal adjustment corrects the problem in many cases.

Captain Nimmo Crepes

Seafood Filling
¾ c. chicken stock
¾ c. white wine
1 onion, chopped
1 lb. shrimp, shelled & deveined
1 lb. crab meat
1 c. sour cream
¾ c. mushrooms, sliced
2 Tbs. butter
1 tsp. lemon juice
½ tsp. salt
¼ tsp. cracked pepper

Crepe Batter
3 large eggs
1½ c. milk
1 c. flour
3 Tbs. butter, melted
2 tsp. brandy
clarified butter

Sauce
3 Tbs. butter
2 Tbs. flour
1½ c. stock (leftover)
4 Tbs. cream
3-4 Tbs. hard cheese, grated

Seafood Filling
Bring stock, wine and onion to a boil, add shrimp and cook 3 minutes. Remove shrimp and save stock. Add crab meat to shrimp; mix in sour cream. Sauté mushrooms in butter and lemon juice; add salt and pepper. Add shellfish to butter mixture and toss well.

Crepes
Put all ingredients in a blender and blend until smooth; let sit one hour. In a 6 - 8" pan, heat a small amount of butter until hot, but not burning. Pour in approximately ¼ c. of batter, roll around bottom of pan to coat and pour off excess. Heat until golden about 30 - 40 seconds; turn over for 10 - 15 seconds. Repeat until finished.

Sauce
Melt butter, add flour, stirring constantly to make a roux. Add stock, cream and cheese slowly until thickened and boiling. Fill crepes with 1½ to 2 tbs. of filling. Roll up and place seam side down in a well buttered baking dish. Cover with sauce. Bake at 400° for approximately 15 minutes until brown and bubbly.

Nimmo: a chiropractic technique. I also like the idea of Captain Nemo from Jules Verne's *20,000 Leagues Under The Sea*.

vegetables & sides

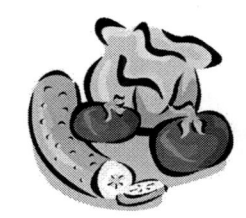

Cervical Collard Greens

2 lbs. collard greens
3 Tbs. olive oil
¼ c. onions, diced
2 cloves garlic, smashed and diced
½ c. tomatoes, diced
¼ c. water
salt and pepper to taste

Wash greens and cut off stems. Heat oil in large skillet, sauté onions and garlic for 2 minutes over medium heat. Add tomatoes and greens, toss and cover. Cook greens for 12 to 15 minutes over low heat or until tender. If greens are drying out, add water, then salt and pepper to taste.

Serves 4.

Cervical collar: a neck support. Certain chiropractic techniques use the neck collar to relax the tension on the spinal column and restore the neck curve. Sometimes a collar is used to prevent much motion when the neck is painful (for example, after an accident).

Vertebrussel Sprouts

1 lb. brussel sprouts
water
salt
¼ c. butter, melted
¼ c. walnuts, chopped or halved
zest from ½ orange

Cut stems off sprouts. Make an X with a small sharp knife in each bottom to promote even cooking. Add to salted water, cook 6 minutes until tender. Drain sprouts, add butter and walnuts. Toss to coat and top with orange zest.

Serves 4 - 6.

Vertebra – a spinal bone. Comes from the Latin word vertere meaning to turn. All vertebrates have vertebrae. Our vertebrae turn and move and that's why we can do yoga. Your vertebrae stack up along your back and your spinal cord lies within the canal created by all the lined-up vertebrae. In fact it's called the spinal canal. Your vertebrae have a body, an arch, joint surfaces, transverse processes, spinous processes and lots of other things chiropractic students have to learn about.

Cervicaliflower and Cheese

1 head cauliflower
⅓ c. butter
⅓ c. flour
1¼ c. milk
1 c. light cream
¼ tsp. white or black pepper
¾ c. cheddar, grated (or other hard cheese)

Wash and trim cauliflower. Cook whole in large pot of water until just tender, about 10 minutes. Drain and place on serving dish. Melt butter, stir in flour to make a roux. Slowly add milk, then cream, stirring constantly to avoid lumps. Cook over low heat until sauce thickens and is smooth. Season sauce with pepper and add cheese. Stir mixture until cheese is melted and thoroughly incorporated. Pour over warm cauliflower.

Serves 6.

Cervical refers to neck. Usually it means the neck under your head. But there are a couple of other necks in the human body. There's the neck of the uterus commonly called the cervix, your urinary bladder has a cervix and even your nerves have a cervix (the axon, for you science nerds.) The neck under your head is made up of seven vertebrae (bones) plus discs, ligaments, tendons, glands and other fancy stuff.

Whiplashed Potatoes with Pinched Herbes

6 medium potatoes
½ c. light cream, heated
3 Tbs. butter
1 tsp. Dijon mustard
1 Tbs. parsley, chopped
1 tsp. chives, chopped
¼ c. parmesan cheese, grated (optional)
salt and pepper to taste

Peel potatoes and cook in boiling water until tender. Drain and mash. Add remaining ingredients and, if you like, a pinch of this and a pinch of that!

Serves 4 - 6.

Whiplash: an acceleration, deceleration injury. Huh? That's when you're moving fast in one direction and then get slammed and the car stops but your head keeps going and then it snaps back. Ugh! A spot of bad news.

Pinched nerves. It used to be said that subluxations pinch nerves. With newer advances in neurophysiology and neuroanatomy that term is no longer used. Nerves are stretched, compressed, irritated, impinged and mechanically altered. What's in a name? Confusion. We have more names but still don't know exactly how a subluxation does so many things. ligaments, tendons, glands and other fancy stuff.

Schmorl's Nodes

2 Tbs. olive oil
12 morel mushrooms, wiped and diced
½ c. onion, minced
1 clove garlic, minced
2 Tbs. parsley, minced
¼ c. water or white wine
pepper to taste
¼ c. parmesan cheese, grated
18 large, fresh white button mushrooms
½ c. butter, melted

Heat oil in skillet. Sauté diced musnrooms, onions, garlic and parsley. Add water or wine, sauté 5 minutes. Add pepper to taste. Remove from heat to cool. Add parmesan cheese and mix. Remove stems from white mushrooms and brush off to remove any dirt. Fill each mushroom cavity with mixture. Place in buttered shallow baking pan. Drizzle with melted butter. Bake at 350° for 20 to 25 minutes.

Serves 4.

Schmorl's Nodes. Sounds like an old vaudeville routine but it's really a form of spinal disease where pieces of your spinal disc, instead of sticking out the side or the back giving you a herniation, decide to do something crazy and stick into the vertebrae above or below. Also called Schmorl nodules.

Praktos Latkes

peanut oil
2 c. potatoes, raw and grated
1 medium onion, diced
2 eggs
¼ c. matzo meal
1½ tsp. salt
½ tsp. baking powder
pepper to taste
sour cream or applesauce (optional)

Heat oil in large skillet. Mix together potatoes, onion, eggs, matzo meal, salt, baking powder and pepper. With large tablespoon or serving spoon (for a side dish or with a teaspoon for hors d'oeuvres), drop each latke (pancake) into skillet and flatten in oil. Fry over moderate heat until golden brown and potatoes are cooked through. Keep warm in oven on baking sheet at 325° for up to 1 hour. Serve plain or with sour cream or applesauce.

Serves 2 - 4.

Praktos: D.D. Palmer asked one of his first patients, Rev. Samuel Weed, a Greek and Latin scholar, to help him name his new "hand treatments." Rev. Weed combined two Greek words, Chiros or Kiros for hand and Praktos for done by, and put them together to make Chiropractic – done by hand. Remember to eat latkes (potato pancakes) with apple sauce or (even better) with sour cream (mmmm good).

Diversifried Rice

4 c. cooked rice, chilled
2 Tbs. oil, peanut or vegetable
2 Tbs. soy sauce
1 egg, beaten
¼ c. diced green onion
½ c. frozen or fresh peas
¼ c. red bell pepper, chopped
¼ c. water chestnuts, chopped
¼ c. bamboo shoots
1 c. chicken, cooked and diced (optional)
½ c. shrimp, diced or use whole baby shrimp (optional)

Heat oil in large skillet or wok. Add rice, soy sauce and stir quickly to coat. Add beaten egg quickly and stir again. When egg is stirred through and appears golden yellow, add remaining ingredients, stirring after each one. If rice gets too dry, add a little water and a few drops of soy sauce. Mixture should be golden brown.

Serves 6 - 8.

The **diversified** chiropractic adjusting procedure is really a hodgepodge of a number of chiropractic techniques. Its most identifiable feature is that it often makes a noise, the pop sound of a joint release. Other techniques, especially those using light touch and those using adjusting instruments, don't make those kind of noises.

Zucchini Foramina Fromagina

2 large zucchini
8 oz. mozzarella, shredded
4 oz. parmesan cheese, grated
1 clove garlic, crushed
¼ c. bread crumbs
2 Tbs. olive oil
4 tomatoes
1 onion
1 green pepper
1 tsp. oregano
salt and pepper to taste

Steam zucchini for about 10 minutes, until just tender. Cool. Cut in half lengthwise. Gently spoon out inside meat leaving a generous border. Mix cheeses, garlic and bread crumbs together. Spoon onto each zucchini half. Oil bottom of baking dish, place zucchini on top. Dice tomatoes, onion and green pepper. Arrange around zucchini, sprinkle with oregano, salt and pepper. Cover with foil. Bake at 350° for about 40 minutes.

Serves 4.

Foramen. A foramen is a hole. Chiropractors are concerned with the little hole or foramina formed when spinal bones (vertebrae) stack up. Nerve roots come out of the spinal cord and go through that spinal foramina to create a spinal nerve that travels all over your body.

Spondylitis Onionitis

4 large yellow onions
½ lb. ground lean hamburger or turkey
¼ c. onions, minced (use centers)
½ c. Italian bread crumbs
1½ Tbs. parsley, minced
2 cloves garlic, crushed
¼ tsp. salt
2 Tbs. parmesan cheese, grated

Peel onions, slice about ¼" off the top of each onion. Cook bottoms in boiling water for about 10 minutes until just barely tender, cool. Remove only the centers, leaving at least ½" of shell. Save centers for stuffing mixture. Mix together ground meat, minced onions, bread crumbs, parsley, garlic and salt. Stuff each shell, place in baking dish and cover with foil. Bake at 400° for 30 minutes. Uncover, top with cheese and bake 10 more minutes.

Serves 4 (or 2 when served as an entree).

Spondylitis: an inflammation of the spine. A vertebral subluxation complex can create spinal inflammation.

Potatoes o'HIO

2 large sweet potatoes
1 Tbs. butter
1 oz. grand marnier
2 Tbs. brown sugar
¼ c. golden raisins
¼ c. pecans, crushed
1 Tbs. orange zest

Bake sweet potatoes about 1 hour at 350°. Cool 10 minutes. Remove meat from shells and mash with butter, grand marnier and sugar. Add raisins and blend. Place in baking dish, sprinkle with nuts and orange zest. Bake at 350° for 30 minutes.

Serves 4.

HIO. Hole-in-one or whole-in-one is a chiropractic analysis and adjusting technique that concentrates on the vertebrae at the top of the spine just below the head – the atlas (C-1). The number of nerve fibers there is astronomical. B.J. Palmer's and others' research on the HIO technique is still being studied.

Nerve Rootabaga

1 large rutabaga
1 tsp. sugar
3 Tbs. butter
¼ tsp. pepper
½ c. parmesan cheese, shredded

Dice rutabaga, cover with water and sugar. Boil for 30 to 35 minutes until tender. Drain. Mash; add butter and pepper. Top with parmesan cheese. Broil for 2-3 minutes.

Serves 4.

Nerve root. Well, nerves gotta come from somewhere. A bunch of rootlets come out of the spinal cord and get together and form a nerve root. Then the nerve root joins more nerves and forms bigger nerves. Then the nerves get together to form a plexus, complexus and gigaplexes. We're all so very complicated, that's why doctors like to consult.

Prolapsed Pintos and Peas

1 lb. pinto beans, picked over
6 c. water
1 clove garlic, minced
¼ c. butter, melted
1 tsp. salt
1 onion, chopped
3 Tbs. molasses
¼ c. ketchup
1 tsp. dry mustard
½ tsp. ground ginger
1½ tsp. Worcestershire sauce
2 Tbs. brown sugar
1 c. fresh or frozen peas

Cover beans with water; bring to a boil for 2 minutes. Still covered, let sit for 1 hour. Add garlic and onion, simmer until tender. Drain, reserving liquid. To liquid add next 8 ingredients, all but peas. Stir and place beans and liquid mixture in a 2 qt. baking dish. Bake in preheated 400° oven for 50 minutes. Carefully remove dish, add peas, stir and bake another 10 minutes.

Serves 6.

A **prolapsed disc** is a very unhappy disc. You could feel really bad. However, in some people with prolapsed disc, there's no pain at all. Go figure.

Toftness Tofu

1 lb. tofu, cut in strips
4 Tbs. soy sauce
2 tsp. corn starch
⅛ tsp. pepper
4 Tbs. peanut oil
4 green peppers, cut in strips
1 c. bamboo shoots, sliced
salt to taste

Mix tofu with 2 Tbs. soy sauce, cornstarch and pepper. Fry in 3 Tbs. oil. Remove after 3 or 4 minutes. Add 1 Tbs. oil and sauté peppers and bamboo shoots. Add remaining soy sauce and tofu. Toss to heat. Add salt if needed.

Serves 4 - 6.

I.N. Toftness, D.C. developed the low force technique that bears his name. Using a set of lenses the doctor can determine where your nerves are being irritated. It is a fascinating study and the Toftness Foundation is making unique contributions to neurophysiology.

Risotto

4 Tbs. butter
1 small onion, minced
1 small clove garlic, minced
1½ c. rice
3½ c. chicken stock (reserving 2 Tbs.)
½ c. white wine
¼ c. butter
1 tsp. saffron
3 Tbs. parmesan cheese, grated

In a saucepan, melt butter, sauté onion and garlic until slightly browned. Stir in rice, add stock and wine; bring to a boil. Cover, let simmer for 25 minutes, stirring often. Soften saffron in 2 Tbs. stock, add ¼ c. butter. Stir then add to rice. Cook rice, uncovered, over low heat for 6 minutes. Place in serving dish and sprinkle with cheese.

Serves 4 - 6.

SOT is short for sacral occipital technique. It's a fascinating method of spinal analysis and adjusting developed by Dr. Major Dejarnette, a gifted thinker and creative scientist.

Koren Pudding

1 Tbs. butter, melted
2 eggs, beaten
1 Tbs. sugar
1 tsp. salt
⅛ tsp. pepper
1 Tbs. flour
¼ c. warm milk
1 can creamed corn
½ c. fresh or whole corn

Mix butter, eggs, sugar, salt, pepper, flour and mil. Pour into a well butter baking dish and bake at 325° for 45 - 50 minutes, until set and golden.

Serves 4.

Two of **Dr. Tedd Koren's** younger brothers are M.D.s. But he takes it in stride. "What the hell," says Koren, "every family's got a black sheep or two."

Achilles Heals

4 baked potatoes (cooled and quartered)
oil for frying
salt and paprika
crisp diced bacon (optional)
sour cream and chives (optional)
melted cheese (optional)

Scoop out potato quarters, leaving enough potato so it keeps firm and skin remains in tact. Save extra potato for potato salad. Heat oil in deep skillet or pot. Fry quarters until browned and crisp, about 8 minutes. Remove and drain on paper towels. Sprinkle with salt and paprika. Serve hot, alone or with bacon, cheese or sour cream and chives.

Serves 4.

Healing: to make whole. No, Achilles wasn't a chiropractor. Enjoy it and tell me some ways we can make it sound more chiropractic-like. Warning – you will not get any money for this idea.

Strained Grains and Bowties

2 c. chicken or beef broth
1 c. medium grain kasha
1 Tbs. butter
½ tsp. salt
¼ tsp. pepper
8 oz. pkg. bowties
water for boiling
1½ Tbs. butter

In small saucepan, heat broth. In medium to large skillet, toast kasha for 2 minutes on medium to high heat, stirring constantly. Reduce heat to low and slowly add hot liquid, butter, salt and pepper. Cover, simmer for 10 minutes until tender. Prepare bowties as directed on package. Strain off liquid and add bowties to kasha. Add butter and toss gently.

Serves 4 - 6.

Strains – another terrible thing we can do to our muscles. A strain is when a muscle becomes overstretched and tears. This painful injury, also called a "pulled muscle," can be caused by an accident, improper use of a muscle or overuse of a muscle.

Crookneck Squash

2 Tbs. olive oil
1 Tbs. fresh basil, chopped
1 Tbs. fresh oregano, chopped
1 clove garlic, chopped
¼ tsp. salt
⅛ tsp. pepper
4 yellow crookneck squash
1 pt. cherry tomatoes

In a small bowl, combine oil with herbs, salt and pepper. Slice squash in half lengthwise and pat dry. Marinate with herbed oil for 1 hour. In hot pan or on grill, cook squash for 4 minutes on cut side. Turn over, add cherry tomatoes and cook 3 - 4 minutes more until just tender.

Serves 4.

Crooked neck. Have you ever seen those squash? They really look like that.

yAKetty yAK yams

3 golden delicious or Granny Smith apples, peeled and cored
3 Tbs. butter
¼ c. firmly packed brown sugar
4 yams, cooked, drained and peeled
1 tsp. orange zest
2 Tbs. maple syrup
¼ c. pecans

Slice apples and sauté in butter 5 minutes, just until tender. Add brown sugar. Stir often. Mash cooked yams, add zest, juice and syrup. Beat until fluffy. Spread mixture in 9" pan or baking dish. Arrange apples on top. Sprinkle with pecans. Pour any remaining butter and sugar syrup over apples. Bake in 350° oven for 15 minutes.

Serves 4.

AK, or **Applied Kinesiology**, is a fascinating analysis technique developed by Dr. George Goodheart. It is sometimes called muscle testing. It's a neuromuscular reflex that is used to evaluate normal and abnormal body function.

Webster's Wee Ones

1 lb. assorted baby squash
1 can baby corn
1 pt. cherry tomatoes
2 Tbs. olive oil
1 Tbs. basil, chopped
1 Tbs. oregano, chopped
1 clove garlic, chopped
salt and pepper to taste

Rinse and pat dry squash. Trim any stems or unsightly bruises. Drain corn. Wash and pat dry tomatoes, remove any stems.

Heat oil in large fry pan. Add vegetables and saute on medium heat for 3 minutes or until squash is tender but firm. Add herbs and garlic. Saute another 2 - 3 minutes. Season with salt and pepper and serve. Great over pasta or rice.

Serves 4 - 6.

The late **Larry Webster, D.C.**, the grandfather of chiropractic pediatrics, is sorely missed by so many of us. A sophisticated intelligence in a down to earth, country doctor personality. Few who knew him were untouched by his warmth, wit and caring. His Webster Breech Technique turned breech presentation babies so they could be delivered naturally, thus saving many women from having caesarean sections.

Ohm's Baby Carrots with Currants

1½ lb. baby carrots
2 Tbs. unsalted butter
2 Tbs. firmly packed light brown sugar
⅓ c. dried currants
salt & fresh ground black pepper

Bring a large pot of lightly salted water to a boil over high heat. Add the baby carrots and cook until barely tender, about 5 minutes. Drain, rinse under cold water and drain again, well. Melt the butter in a large skillet over medium heat, add the carrots, brown sugar and ¼ cup water. Cook, stirring often, until the carrots are heated through and the liquid has evaporated into a glaze, about 5 minutes. Stir in the currants, season with salt and pepper. Transfer to a serving dish and serve hot.

Serves 8.

Ohm – a unit of electrical resistance equal to that of a conductor in which a current (current, currants – get it?) of one ampere is produced by a potential of one volt across its terminals.

OK, really. **Jeanne Ohm, D.C.** is the high-voltage executive director of the International Chiropractic Pediatric Association (www.icpa4kids.com), an organization that provides education, training and support research on chiropractic care in pregnancy and throughout childhood because all children need chiropractic care. It's one of the most exciting organizations in the entire chiropractic

Masters Circle Power Rings

8 large onions
1½ c. flour
4 Tbs. cornmeal
4 Tbs. onion powder
2 tsp. salt
1½ c. milk
1 large egg
½ c. water
oil for frying

Combine flour, cornmeal, onion powder, salt, milk, egg and water in large mixing bowl. Stir well until there are no lumps. Slice onions about ½" thick and separate into rings. Dip rings into batter. Drop rings into deep fryer or 3" deep oil in large pan and cook until golden brown. Drain on paper towels and serve.

Serves 8.

The Masters Circle has become one of the most well respected and best known Leadership Training and Practice Building organizations. Drs. Bob Hoffman, Dennis Perman and Larry Markson have created an "identity based" organization, emphasizing that the true power and success in chiropractic practice comes from knowing who you are and being committed to the unique healing that chiropractic offers.

breads

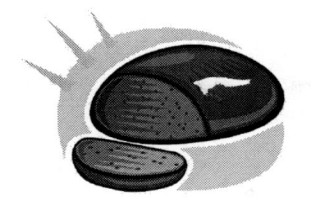

Koren Bread

3 c. whole wheat flour
1 c. flour
2 tsp. salt
1 tsp. baking soda
1 tsp. baking powder
1 Tbs. dill
1¾ c. buttermilk

Sift together dry ingredients, add dill. Mix in buttermilk to make a soft but firm dough. Knead on floured surface for 3 minutes until smooth. Make a round loaf and put in a greased 8" cake pan or on a cookie sheet. Make an X on top with a knife. Bake at 375° for 40 minutes, or until browned and hollow-sounding (using your knuckles, rap on top). Cool, then slice.

Tedd Koren, D.C. loves spicy food but his wife doesn't. When they go to Indian restaurants he orders no spice so they can share. What a guy!

Spoondylitis Bread

1½ c. milk
1 can cream of asparagus soup
1 c. yellow cornmeal
4 eggs, separated
2 Tbs. butter, melted
½ c. asparagus tips (parboiled and cooled)

Mix together milk and soup, add cornmeal. Cook slowly, stirring constantly until it looks like mush. Beat egg yolks, add butter and stir into cornmeal mixture. Beat egg whites until stiff peak stage (not dry) and fold into mixture. Add asparagus, folding gently. Bake in buttered dish or casserole at 350° for 1 hour. Top should be tender and springy when touched.

Serves 4.

Spondylitis: inflammation of the vertebrae. It's very common when you have a subluxation.

Snap Crackle Popovers

butter
3 eggs
1½ c. milk
1½ c. flour
½ tsp. salt
½ tsp. dill or crushed rosemary
1½ Tbs. oil

Preheat oven to 475°. Heavily butter 8 large muffin tins, ceramic or glass cups. Combine eggs, milk, flour, salt and dill or rosemary. Using a blender or mixer, beat until smooth, about 2 minutes. Add oil to batter and beat for 20 seconds. Fill cups halfway. Place on baking sheet on bottom rack of oven and bake 15 minutes. Lower temperature to 350° - DO NOT OPEN OVEN DOOR - and continue baking 25 minutes until golden and set. Poke muffins with a fork. Turn off heat and leave muffins in oven another 20 minutes.

Serves 8.

Snap, crackle, pop. No, no, chiropractors adjust. They don't snap, crack or pop spines or bones. Who put this title in here anyway? Heads will roll. Call a staff meeting...

Flexion Bread

1 pkg. active dry yeast
2 Tbs. sugar
1½ c. warm water
5 c. flour (quantity depending on weather)
2 tsp. salt
2 eggs
2 Tbs. oil
1 egg yolk
2 Tbs. sesame seeds

Mix yeast and sugar in ¼ c. warm water. Let sit for 5 minutes. Sift flour with salt in a large bowl. Make a hole in the center of the flour. Place eggs, oil and rest of water in the hole. Work flour into the liquids a little at a time. When combined, turn out onto a floured board or surface. Knead dough until smooth. Make a ball and place in a lightly greased bowl, greasing ball all over. Cover and let rise 1 hour. Punch down, cover and let double approximately 1½ hours. Divide into three parts. Flour hands and roll each part into a rope. Braid the three ropes. Place on a greased cookie sheet. Bring the ends around until almost touching, like a horseshoe. Cover and let rise again until doubled. Brush with egg yolk and sprinkle with sesame seeds. Bake at 375° for 45 minutes until golden brown.

Flexion, extension, lateral flexion and extension, these are some of the ways your body moves. When you flex you bring two body parts closer together – like when you flex your muscles the parts your muscles are connected to come closer together. Extension is the opposite. People are asked to flex and extend body parts, especially their neck and hips, as part of range of motion tests.

My Grains Bread

¼ c. warm water
1 pkg. active dry yeast
1 Tbs. sugar
1½ c. hot water
3 Tbs. butter
¼ c. brown sugar, firmly packed
1½ tsp. salt
2 c. whole wheat flour
¾ c. wheat germ
2 c. unbleached flour, sifted
¼ c. sunflower seeds, unsalted
2 Tbs. poppy seeds

In warm water, soften yeast and sugar for 5 minutes. Mix hot water with butter, brown sugar and salt, set aside for 5 minutes. Stir in wheat flour, wheat germ and half of white flour. Mix well. Stir in yeast and seeds. Keep blending until almost stiff, adding more white flour as needed. Turn out onto floured board. Knead 10 minutes, until smooth. Shape into a ball and place in a greased bowl, grease dough and cover. Let rise until doubled, 1 to 2 hours. Punch down and cut in half. Shape into 2 balls. Cover and let dough relax for 15 minutes. Shape into loaves in well greased pans. Cover again and let rise 1 to 2 hours more. Bake at 375° for 45 minutes, until crusty and they sound hollow when tapped.

Migraines. It technically refers to a severe kind of head pain that is on one side of the head, with nausea, vomiting and other disturbances. Anyone suffering from migraines should see a chiropractor to get their subluxations corrected.

desserts & sweets

Chocolate Torticollis

1 lb. German's sweet chocolate
1 tsp. Grand Marnier
½ c. butter, room temperature
5 large eggs, separated
cocoa (powdered)
¼ c. confectionary sugar
raspberries

Preheat oven to 250° degrees. Grease springform pan and dust with cocoa. Melt chocolate with butter. In a large bowl mix egg yolks and Grand Marnier with a fork. Slowly beat warm melted chocolate into yolks until blended. In small bowl beat whites until stiff, and slowly add confectionary sugar. Fold whites into chocolate mixture ⅓ at a time. Bake for 1 hour until toothpick thrust into top of torte comes out almost clean. Cool torte in pan. Cut into 12 wedges. Alternating, dust every other wedge with cocoa and then confectionary sugar. Garnish with raspberries.

Serves 12.

Torticollis. It's when your neck is twisted to one side and you can't straighten it out and it really, really hurts.

Sacrumb Cake

½ c. butter
1 c. sugar
2 eggs
1½ tsp. vanilla
2 c. flour
1 tsp. baking powder
1 tsp. baking soda
2 tsp. poppy seeds (optional)
1 tsp. cinnamon
dash nutmeg
dash salt
1 c. sour cream

Topping

½ c. brown sugar
1 tsp. cinnamon
2 Tbs. butter, melted

Cream together butter and sugar. Add eggs and vanilla, beat well. Sift together flour, baking powder and soda, cinnamon, nutmeg and salt. Add to creamed mixture alternately with sour cream. Add poppy seeds. Spread batter in a greased 13" x 9" x 2" baking pan. Combine topping ingredients and sprinkle over batter. Bake at 350° for 35 - 40 minutes.

Sacrum. It's at the bottom of your spine. It's shaped like a pyramid. Hmm, I wonder if that's where pyramid power comes from?

Scolioatmeal Cookie Logs

1 c. butter, melted
½ c. quick cooking oats
1 c. brown sugar
½ c. sifted flour
4 Tbs. cream
12 oz. chocolate chips, melted
½" or 1" wooden dowel (can use broom stick)

Combine all ingredients except chocolate. Cook over medium heat, stirring constantly until it begins to bubble. Remove from heat and drop by rounded teaspoonfuls onto greased and floured cookie sheet, 4 - 5 inches apart (no more than 6 per sheet). Bake at 375° for 5 minutes until golden. Let sit for ½ minute then carefully remove and place over dowel (wrapping loosely) until cool and firm. When all cookies are finished and cooled, dip ⅓ of each cookie in chocolate. Place on wax paper until firm.

Makes 24 - 30 cookies.

Scoliosis is when your spine is crooked sideways. Most everyone's spine is a teeny bit crooked here or there but some people with scoliosis can have a spine that's extremely distorted to the side. Most scoliotics can live normal lives, birth children and go about their business. The cause of scoliosis is a big mystery.

Energy Cookie Bars

3 eggs
1 c. honey
1½ tsp. vanilla
1½ c. sifted flour
1 tsp. baking powder
1 c. Turkish apricots, diced
1 c. pitted dates, diced
1 c. pecans, chopped
1 c. coconut

Beat eggs until light. Add honey and vanilla, beat again. Stir in flour, baking powder, apricots, dates, pecans and coconut. Bake in a greased 13" x 9" x 2" pan at 350° for 45 minutes. Cool; cut into finger length bars and roll in coconut.

Makes approximately 3 dozen bars.

Energy. Life energy is described in many different cultures: vital force, prana, ch'i. As scientific instruments become more sensitive, subtler levels of energy are detected within us and in the Universe.

Triune Prune Pastry

2 c. sifted flour
2 tsp. baking powder
dash salt
½ c. butter
1 tsp. orange zest, chopped fine
1 c. sugar
1 egg
1 Tbs. orange juice
1 Tbs. Grand Marnier
1 jar lekvar (prune butter)
water

Sift together dry ingredients. Cream butter and orange zest together. Gradually add sugar. Beat until fluffy; add egg, orange juice and Grand Marnier. Beat well; add dry ingredients to mixture to make a soft dough. Chill. Roll out onto floured board ⅛" thick. Cut into rounds using a floured glass rim. Put 1 tsp. of lekvar in the center of each circle. Bring up the edges to form a triangle. Moisten with water to form a good seal. Bake at 400° on ungreased cookie sheets for 10 to 12 minutes, until just barely golden. Do not overbake.

Makes 15 - 20.

Triune of Life – energy, intelligence and matter. Ever wonder how your thoughts convert into physical activities? Let's say you think about raising your hand and then you raise your hand. Where was that place where your non-material thought became a physical action? No one knows. It's truly something to wonder about. The Triune of Life discusses that phenomenon.

Chocolate Wave Zucchini Bread

⅓ c. butter
1⅓ c. sugar
2 eggs
1½ c. grated zucchini
⅓ c. water
1 tsp. vanilla
1⅔ c. flour
1 tsp. baking soda
½ tsp. salt
¼ tsp. baking powder
1 tsp. pumpkin pie spice
⅓ c. chopped walnuts
3 Tbs. unsweetened cocoa powder
⅓ c. mini semi-sweet chocolate chips

Preheat oven to 350°. Grease one 9" x 5" loaf pan. In a large bowl, cream butter and sugar together. Mix in eggs. Add zucchini, water, and vanilla; stir. Blend in flour, baking soda, salt, baking powder, and pumpkin pie spice. Stir in nuts.

Divide batter in half, and add cocoa powder and chocolate chips to one of the halves. Pour plain batter into bottom of the loaf pan. Pour chocolate batter on top of plain batter. Bake until wooden pick inserted into center comes out clean, about 1 hour. Cool 10 minutes, and remove from pan. Store in refrigerator.

Serves 12.

Eat this dessert after you see your NSA (Network Spinal Analysis) doctor. Donald Epstein, D.C., developer of NSA, teaches doctors all over the world to make their patients wave. **Wave?** The Network wave, a powerful stress releaser, is a physiological phenomenon that involves your entire body waving or undulating as you release stress. The wave goes from your head to your hips to your toes and feels great!

Chiro Crunch Cookies

¼ lb. butter
1 c. light brown sugar, packed
1 egg, large
½ tsp. vanilla
1 c. chunky peanut butter
1½ c. flour, sifted
1 tsp. baking soda
2 Tbs. bran
4 oz. peanut butter chips

Cream together butter and sugar, add egg and vanilla. Add peanut butter and beat again. Sift flour and baking soda, add to butter mixture. Beat again; add bran and chips. Chill at least 4 hours or overnight. Preheat oven to 350°. Form dough into 1½" balls, press down lightly with palm of hand. Use a fork to decorate the edges if you like. Bake 10 minutes; cool.

Makes approximately 4 dozen cookies.

Crunch. One of the great things that low-force techniques and adjusting instruments have given to the profession, apart from their obvious manner of adjusting with little force, is that bone "crunching" is not done. There's no popping or "cracking" sound. The bone cruncher would be a good name for a wrestler.

No Mercy Chocolate Mousse Pie

1 chocolate crumb pie shell
8 oz. semi-sweet chocolate pieces
¼ c. Grand Marnier
5 eggs separated
¼ c. whipping cream

Melt chocolate in Grand Marnier over very low heat or in top of double boiler, stirring constantly. DO NOT BURN. Cool. Separate eggs. One at a time, beat egg yoks into chocolate mixture. Whip the cream and fold into chocolate mixture. Beat egg whites until stiff and gently fold into chocolate. Pile lightly into pie shell. Chill. Pipe on extra whipped cream if desired.

Serves 6.

The **Mercy Document** was a statement put together by a bunch of chiropractors with too much free time on their hands. It was designed to tell everybody how to practice – a great way to tone down creativity. Fortunately it has been largely forgotten.

Grassom Grasshopper Pie

1 8" cookie crumb crust
1 7 oz. jar marshmallow creme
¼ c. green creme de menthe
1 pt. heavy whipping cream
¾ c. peppermint candy, crushed (optional)

Mix marshmallow creme with liqueur until smooth. Whip cream until thick and stiff. Mix into marshmallow mixture. Fold in half the crushed candy. Pour into pie shell. Sprinkle with remainder of candy and freeze.

Serves 6.

Ian Grassom, D.C. was a wonderful speaker. Hear him once and you'd never forget him. Full of fire, passion and wit – give me a hundred like him and hospitals would be converted to macaroni factories.

Big Guy Berry Pie

1 cup water
¾ c. sugar
¼ tsp. salt
2 Tbs. cornstarch
1 c. flour
½ c. butter
3 Tbs. confectioner's sugar
1 tsp. vanilla
1 quart fresh berries (hulled, if strawberries)

In a saucepan, combine water, sugar, salt, and cornstarch. Bring to a boil, and cook for about 5 minutes or until thickened. Set aside to cool. Preheat oven to 350°. In a large bowl, combine flour, butter, confectioners' sugar and vanilla. Mix well and press into a 9" pie pan. Prick all over and bake in preheated oven for 8 to 10 minutes, or until lightly browned. When crust is cool, place berries in the shell, and pour the thickened mixture over the top. Chill in refrigerator. Serve with a dollop of whipped cream.

Serves 6.

Guy Reikeman, D.C. has done it all. First he was my teacher at Sherman College (no mean feat). Than he teamed up with Joe Flesia, D.C. to form Renaissance International, one of the most groundbreaking organizations the profession has ever seen. Reanssiance was into it all: research, philosophy, science, saving the world and educating doctor and patients. Guy then created his own practice management company and, if that weren't enough, became the president of chiropractic colleges. Whew.

Insurance Bluesberry Cobbler

1 egg
¾ c. sugar
3 Tbs. butter, melted
⅓ c. milk
1 tsp. vanilla
½ c. flour, sifted
2 tsp. baking powder
3 c. blueberries, washed and picked over
1 c. sliced peaches
½ tsp. cinnamon

Beat egg with half of the sugar and the melted butter; add milk and vanilla. Sift flour with baking powder. Beat dry ingredients into batter. Mix blueberries and peaches with cinnamon and remaining sugar. Place in a well buttered casserole or baking dish (2 qt. or 12" x 8" pan). Spread batter evenly on top of fruit. Bake at 375° for 35 - 40 minutes, until set and golden brown.

Serves 6.

Insurance blues. Third party payers. Oh, all those forms and terms. You need a degree just to do the paperwork.

TransMission Fig Nut Bread

3½ c. all purpose flour
⅔ c. sugar
1 tsp. salt
4 tsp. baking powder
3 Tbs. butter
1½ c. milk
1 egg, beaten
8 oz. fresh mission figs
4 oz. pistachio or walnut pieces

In a large bowl, stir together dry ingredients. Cut in butter until it looks like crumbs. Stir in milk and egg until blended, do not over mix. Remove stems from figs and slice. Add figs and nuts to batter. Butter a 9" x 5" loaf pan (lined with buttered wax paper) and lightly dust with flour. Pour in batter and bake at 375° for 1 hour, until golden and toothpick comes out clean.

Transmission. It's part of the Triune of Life (see page 145). The wisdom of your body transmits the energy and wisdom of life over your nerves. That's why its so important to keep your nerves healthy.

Sherman Chocolate Cake

Cake
4 oz. Lindt milk chocolate
½ c. warm water
1 c. butter
1¾ c. sugar
3 egg yolks
1 tsp. vanilla
½ tsp. salt
1 tsp. baking soda
2¼ c. cake flour
¾ c. buttermilk
4 egg whites

Frosting
1 c. evaporated milk
¾ c. sugar
3 egg yolks
½ c. butter
1 tsp. vanilla
1 c. chopped pecans
1½ c. shredded coconut

Grease two 9" cake pans, line bottom with wax paper and grease paper. Melt chocolate with water, stir until melted and incorporated. Cool. Beat butter with sugar until fluffy. Add yolks, one at a time, beating well after each one. Add cooled chocolate and vanilla. Sift dry ingredients. Add half of flour mixture to chocolate, then add ½ of buttermilk and repeat, beating until light and smooth. Beat egg whites until stiff, but not dry, and fold into batter. Pour into cake pans. Bake 40 - 50 minutes at 350°, until toothpick inserted in center comes out clean. Cool 15 minutes, then turn out onto wire racks to cool completely.

Mix evaporated milk, sugar, egg yolks, butter and vanilla in large saucepan. Cook until mixture thickens, 10 - 15 minutes. Add pecans, mix well. Add coconut, mix well again. Cool. Spread frosting on tops of layers and place one on top of the other. Traditional German chocolate cake does not have icing around the sides.

Sherman College of Straight Chiropractic was named after Lyle Sherman, D.C. who worked with B.J. Palmer in his world famous research clinic. A warm man with a large heart, he constantly regaled us (students at Sherman) with B.J. stories.

D.D.'s Double Dipped Mint Cookies

½ c. butter
1 c. sugar
2 eggs
1 Tbs. peppermint extract
2 c. sifted flour
2 tsp. baking powder
½ tsp. salt
1 lb. semi sweet chocolate
12 oz. white chocolate

Beat together butter and sugar, add eggs and mint. Sift together dry ingredients and stir into butter mixture. Drop by teaspoonfuls onto ungreased cookie sheet. Bake at 375° for 8 - 10 minutes. Cool on wire racks.

Melt dark chocolate. Quickly dip cooled cookie halfway into chocolate then place on wax paper until completely cooled. Melt white chocolate and dip cookie ⅓ of the way into warm chocolate and again place on wax paper until completely cooled. You can dip one end in dark chocolate and the opposite end in white chocolate or, if you prefer, dip the same side in each chocolate using the cookie as a handle. Looks great either way.

Makes approximately 48 cookies.

Not much is written on what **D.D. Palmer** liked to eat. He sold raspberries and honey at one time so I guess he might have had a fondness for sweets. He also sold goldfish. What does that tell us? Goldfish are a variety of carp. Carp go into gefilte fish. Did D.D. like gefilte fish?

Thoracicles

2 bananas
1 pt. strawberries
1½ c. grapefruit, orange or apple juice
14 - 20 popsicle sticks

Mash fruits. Press through a strainer or sieve. Add juice. Pour mixture into an ice cube tray. Freeze 30 - 60 minutes until almost hard and place a popsicle stick in each section. Freeze 2 - 3 hours longer. Any fruit or juice can be substituted.

Makes 14 - 20 popsicles.

Thoracic: your mid-back. The area where your fibs go. Cute play on words, huh?

Nervana Banana Bread

3 medium ripe bananas
½ c. vegetable oil
1 c. sugar
2 eggs, beaten slightly
2 c. flour
½ tsp. baking powder
1 tsp. baking soda
pinch salt
3 Tbs. milk
1 tsp. vanilla
6 oz. mini chocolate chips

Mash bananas. Beat oil and sugar together, add eggs and bananas. Beat well. Sift together dry ingredients and add to mixture. Add milk and vanilla. Mix well. Stir in chocolate chips. Pour batter into greased and floured 9" x 5" loaf pan or two smaller pans. Bake at 350° for 1 hour to 1 hour 10 minutes or until toothpick inserted in center comes out clean. Freezes well.

Nerve: the cell of communication. A nerve cell is also called a neuron and it's usually long and thin and can send messages all over you. As you read these words millions and billions of nerves are firing across your brain and body. Hey, keep it down will you?

Toggle Toffee

½ c. dark corn syrup
1 c. brown sugar, firmly packed
¼ c. butter
⅓ c. cream
½ tsp. vanilla or almond extract

Mix corn syrup, brown sugar, butter and cream together in a saucepan, bring to a boil. Candy thermometer should read about 280° or hard stage when ready. Stir in extract. Pour into 8" buttered square pan. Cool. Lightly cut or mark into serving squares. When completely cooled, turn out onto a board and break where cuts are indicated.

If you are ambitious, dip each piece in melted chocolate and then into crushed nuts (makes a wonderful gift).

Makes approximately ½ lb. toffee.

A **toggle** is a type of specific chiropractic adjusting technique that takes years of practice to fully master. In the hands of an accomplished doctor it can work miracles.

Loganberry Crepes and Whipped Cream

Crepes

2 eggs
¼ c. milk
¼ c. water
1 Tbs. Grand Marnier
1 Tbs. clarified butter
½ c. flour

¼ tsp. salt
1 Tbs. sugar
½ tsp. vanilla
½ tsp. grated orange zest
extra clarified butter

Put all ingredients in a blender and whirl until smooth with no lumps. Let rest for 30 to 60 minutes.

Filling

2 c. loganberries (or other if not available)
1 Tbs. Grand Marnier
1 c. whipped cream
2-3 Tbs. powdered sugar

Marinate berries in Grand Marnier while making crepes. Whip the cream, add sugar to taste and fold in drained berries.

Heat 6 - 8" sauté pan, wipe with clarified butter. Pour in ¼ cup batter, roll it around in pan and drain off excess. Heat crepe for 30 seconds on each side. Repeat. Put 1 - 2 Tbs. cream mixture in center of each crepe and roll up. Place seam side down on serving platter. Any remaining berry mixture can be served on the side or on top of the crepes.

Serves 4 - 6.

Logan College of Chiropractic was founded by Dr. Vince Logan who is famous for his "basic technique."

Allopathy Taffy

1 c. sugar
½ c. light corn syrup
½ c. water
¾ tsp. salt
1 tsp. glycerine (available at drug stores)
1 Tbs. butter
1 tsp. vanilla, peppermint, almond or orange extract

In a medium saucepan, mix together sugar, corn syrup, water, salt and glycerine. Stir constantly over low heat until it reaches 260° on a candy thermometer. Remove from heat, add butter and flavoring. Pour onto a greased pan or platter. Cool. Grease hands and pull candy until lightly colored and it becomes too hard to pull any more. Stretch it into a long rope (it's useful to have a friend help you at this juncture) about ¼" thick. Cut into 1" pieces. Wrap each piece in candy or wax paper.

Makes approximately ½ lb.

Allopathic medicine: allopaths or regular medical physicians who follow a mechanistic philosophy of healthcare. In the other corner we have an opposing philosophy of healthcare that is practiced by homeopaths, chiropractors, osteopaths, naturopaths and others who have an empirical or vitalistic philosophy. Samuel Hahnemann, M.D. coined the term allopathy for modern medicine, meaning they are all over the place.

National Mixed Fruit Yogurt Pie

8 oz. strawberry yogurt
8 oz. raspberry yogurt
8 oz. Cool Whip
1 graham cracker pie crust, ready made
9 large strawberries
24 blueberries

In medium bowl, mix together yogurts and Cool Whip. Pour into pie crust. Place extra mixture (if any) in separate, freezer-proof container and cover. Decorate top of pie with outer circle of strawberries, placing one in the center, and inner circle of blueberries. Cover and freeze. Defrost for approximately ½ hour before serving. Experiment with other flavors too.

Serves 6 - 8.

National College. Mix is an old term that refers to the mixing of chiropractic or empirical (vitalistic) and medical or mechanistic belief systems. National College is considered by many to mix those two philosophical systems.

Gelardi Gelati

12 oz. ricotta cheese
1½ c. milk
½ c. honey
1 pt. strawberries or blackberries, cleaned, hulled and chopped
1 tsp. vanilla

Puree ricotta until creamy. In a saucepan, add ricotta, milk and honey. Stirring constantly, bring to a boil over medium heat. Add vanilla and berries. On low heat, stir 2 minutes to incorporate berries. Let rest for 10 minutes. Using an ice cream maker, freeze according to directions, or use a metal pan. Freeze until set, covered with plastic wrap. Scoop out and serve. Mixture may need to sit out at room temperature for 5 minutes to make serving easier.

Serves 6.

Thom Gelardi, D.C. is the founder and past president of the Sherman College of Straight Chiropractic.

straights & mixers

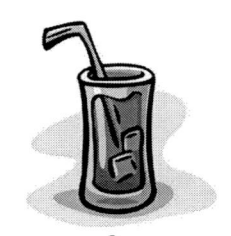

Sigafoose Juice

¾ c. lime juice
1 c. lemon juice
4 tsp. white horseradish
1 tsp. Worcestershire sauce
1 tsp. Tabasco sauce (optional)
1 tsp. salt
1 tsp. pepper
1 Tbs. sugar
1 large can tomato juice

Mix together first 8 ingredients until well blended. Pour in tomato juice and stir.

Makes approximately 2 quarts.

James Sigafoose, D.C. He's had one of the largest, if not the largest, practices in the world – he's done it all. He's a lecturer, traveler, writer, entertainer, philosopher – and he wears Indian hats. He's like a modern day B.J. Palmer. Except that he smiles. What more can a man do?

Centennial Punch

6 c. water
1 orange, thinly sliced
¾ c. superfine sugar
2 bottles sauterne
3 bottles champagne (inexpensive)
½ bottle orange flavored seltzer
1 c. strawberries, sliced

Freeze water in 6 cup ring mold overnight. Place orange slices in a large punch bowl; sprinkle sugar over slices. Add 1 bottle of sauterne; let marinate for an hour or two. Add remaining ingredients; stir gently. Add ice and serve.

Makes approximately 6 quarts.

The **centennial** of the discovery of chiropractic by D.D. Palmer was 1995. There was a big celebration in Davenport, Iowa. It was a lot of fun except there wasn't enough food. I hope they use a different caterer next time.

Liga Mint Julep

4 tsp. sugar
¼ c. water
crushed ice
6 - 8 oz. bourbon, peach brandy or rum
12 sprigs fresh mint

Chill 4 mugs or glasses in freezer for 2 hours. Dissolve sugar in water. Fill glasses with crushed ice. Pour liquor and dissolved sugar into a small pitcher, stir. Pour over crushed ice in frosty glasses, stir again and decorate with mint sprigs. Add straws.

Serves 4.

Ligament. Your gristle. It connects your bones to your bones. Ligaments are a form of connective tissue. Connective tissue connects skin to muscle and muscle to bone. "A mind that's weak and a back that's strong, you dig sixteen tons, what do you get?" A free visit to the chiropractor.

Innate Flash

½ c. sugar
½ c. water
1 cinnamon stick
1 orange, sliced
1 lime, sliced
1 bottle red wine
¼ c. Cointreau
6 oz. orange or lime flavored seltzer

Heat water with sugar to boiling, add cinnamon stick and cook 6 minutes, making a syrup. Add fruit slices and marinate at room temperature for 2 hours. Add wine and Cointreau, stir. Pour into a pitcher, add seltzer and ice.

Serves 6.

In chiropractic philosophy **Innate** (inborn) intelligence refers to the inborn wisdom of your body – your inner healer. "Tuning in to Innate" is what the chiropractic adjustment helps accomplish – it helps connect you to your innate intelligence. An innate flash is a conscious insight into your inner wisdom. Inspiration!

Lack of Coordination

¼ lb. sugar
½ c. lemon juice
2 c. brandy
½ c. dark rum
¼ c. peach schnapps or brandy
ice
1 peach

Dissolve sugar in lemon juice; add rest of ingredients. Use sliced peach for garnish; add ice and serve.

Makes approximately 1 quart.

Coordination is the harmonious functioning of interrelated organs or parts. For optimal health, for the proper adaptation to your environment, all your internal organs, glands, and muscles must work together in a coordinated manner. That is done under the direction of your inner wisdom using your brain, spinal cord and nerves. The vertebral subluxation complex damages the nervous system and causes lack of coordination. Warning: this drink may cause lack of coordination, too.

T4 Two

2 qts. water
4 cinnamon sticks
10 whole cloves
6 tea bags
1½ c. sugar
2 lemons, juiced
1 orange, juice and rind
1 Tbs. Grand Marnier or peach schnapps

Boil water with cinnamon and cloves for 10 minutes. Add tea bags, lemon and orange juice and liqueur, cook for 10 more minutes. Remove from heat, add orange rind and cool at room temperature. Discard bags and rind. Pour over ice and adjust sugar to taste.

Makes 2 quarts.

T4 is a way of writing fourth thoracic vertebrae. Your 24 vertebrae are named using a simple formula. Your twelve thoracic vertebrae are named T1, T2, T3, to T12. Your cervical vertebrae are named C1 to C7; your lumbars are L1 to L5. The nerves that come out between T3 and T4 and T4 and T5 go to your lungs, heart, gallbladder and bronchial tubes, among others.

Fountainhead Froth

2 c. milk
1 tsp. vanilla
1 large ripe banana
8 large strawberries

Put milk in freezer for about 10 minutes, until icy cold. Blend milk with vanilla, banana and 6 strawberries until frothy. Pour into large glasses. Cut each of remaining strawberries almost in half vertically and place on rim of glass.

Serves 2.

Fountainhead: The source; the mother load. Traditionally this refers to the Palmer College of Chiropractic, founded by the Founder of Chiropractic, D.D. Palmer.

Cloud Walker

1 oz. Lapponia Lakka Cloudberry Liqueur
¾ oz. Johnnie Walker Scotch Whiskey
⅓ oz. lime juice
2 oz. lemonade

Pour into an old-fashioned glass filled with broken ice. Add a lime slice, and serve.

Serves 1.

You lost your dog at age 4 and that's causing your subluxation to recur? Your mother yelled at you when you were 6 and now your body is not working right? Using **Scott Walker, D.C.**'s Neuro Emotional Technique (NET) you can find that out. What is NET? It's a technique that releases deep emotional stress (neuro emotional complexes or NECs) from old emotional traumas. Using a combination of acupuncture, muscle testing and chiropractic, old chronic subluxations suddenly start holding, phobias begin to fade away, even writer's block clears up. People do seem to be walking on clouds after they get adjusted.

Fixation

1 qt. apple cider
½ bottle Applejack Brandy
2 cinnamon sticks
6 cloves, whole
1 tsp. ground ginger
1 tsp. nutmeg
sugar (if needed)

Simmer ingredients in large pot for 15 minutes. Remove cinnamon sticks and cloves. Add sugar if needed. Serve hot or cold.

Serves 6.

A joint is normally able to move in a variety of different directions or range of motion. But, when there's a **fixation** present, the joint is locked in at least one direction. For example, you can turn your head to the right, but not as much to the left (it's fixated on the left) or lower your head but not raise it. Fixation is one of the components of the subluxation complex. Technically, when a joint is locked or fixated it causes your nerves to fire in an unusual manner (abnormal afferent sensory-bed disturbance). That upsets your spinal cord and all kinds of spinal cord reflexes shoot out that can affect the internal organs, muscles and higher neurological centers including your brain.

Motion Pulpation Spritzers

16 oz. orange juice with pulp, chilled
10 large strawberries
1 tsp. vanilla (optional)
16 oz. club soda, chilled

In blender, mix together juice with 6 berries and vanilla. Add club soda and pour into 4 serving glasses. Garnish each with a strawberry.

Serves 4.

The chiropractors of Belgium did not have access to X-ray and Dr. Henri Gillet of Belgium developed **motion palpation** to overcome this limitation. Using motion palpation the patient's vertebrae and hips are tested by moving them in different directions to find if they're locked. It has been popularized in North America by Leonard Faye, D.C. of Canada.

Range of Motion Potion

6 oz. orange juice
6 oz. pear nectar
6 oz. peach nectar
6 oz. pineapple juice
8 strawberries
8 ice cubes
4 pineapple spears or orange slices

Mix juices, strawberries and ice cubes in blender until smooth, about 1 minute. Pour into 4 glasses. Garnish with fresh fruit.

Serves 4.

Range of motion tells you how well your parts move. Didn't I already tell you this?

Degeneration

1 bottle sparking apple juice, chilled
3 oz. apple brandy
1 tsp. cinnamon
½ tsp. nutmeg
1 apple, cored and quartered
1 tsp. lemon juice
ice cubes

Mix juice, brandy, cinnamon and nutmeg in a 1½ to 2 quart pitcher. Pour over ice cubes into glasses. Coat apple wedges with lemon juice and place one on each glass as garnish.

Serves 4.

Degeneration. It's done by aliens with ray guns. Oh, that's disintegration. Degeneration is a slow process of accelerated aging and wasting away that happens when you're full of subluxations, referred to as subluxation degeneration. Not a good thing to have. Regular chiropractic adjustments can help reverse spinal or subluxation degeneration.

Clear View Carrot Juice

1 qt. carrot juice
1 tsp. curry powder
1 Tbs. parsley, chopped
1 Tbs. green onion, chopped
hot sauce to taste (optional)

Boil carrot juice 2 minutes, skim off solids and foam, discard. Add curry powder. Chill broth. Pour into 4 glasses. Top with parsley and green onions. Add a dash of hot sauce if desired.

Serves 4.

Clear View Sanitarium was operated by chiropractors for the care of the mentally ill. Along with Forest Park and many other similar institutions chiropractors got better results caring for the mentally ill than the state mental hospitals did using only medical care which included electric shock therapy, frontal lobotomies and drugs. It's time for a re-birth of these institutions.

Glossary

bain marie ....a pan of hot water with a smaller dish or pan inside

baste................... to moisten (meat, for example) periodically with a liquid, such as melted butter or a sauce, especially while cooking

braise ....to cook (meat or vegetables) by browning in fat, then simmering in a small quantity of liquid in a covered container

chop ....cut into small pieces

clarified butter...butter made clear by heating and removing the sediment of milk solids

dice.....................cut into small cubes

grate....................to reduce to fragments, shreds or powder by rubbing against an abrasive surface

knead ....to mix and work into a uniform mass, as by folding, pressing and stretching with the hands

mince ....cut or chop into very small pieces

roux ....a mixture of flour and fat cooked together and used as a thickening

sauté...................to fry lightly in fat in a shallow open pan

sinew.................. a tendon

Measurements

a pinch	⅛ teaspoon or less
3 teaspoons	1 tablespoon
4 tablespoons	¼ cup
8 tablespoons	½ cup
12 tablespoons	¾ cup
16 tablespoons	1 cup
2 cups	1 pint
4 cups	1 quart
4 quarts	1 gallon
16 ounces	1 pound
32 ounces	1 quart
1 ounce liquid	2 tablespoons
8 ounces liquid	1 cup

Use standard measuring spoons and cups. All measurements are level.

Substitutions

Ingredient	Quantity	Substitute
baking powder	1 teaspoon	¼ tsp. baking soda plus ½ tsp. cream of tartar
catsup or chili sauce	1 cup	1 c. tomato sauce plus ½ cup sugar and 2 T. vinegar (for use in cooking)
chocolate	1 square (1 oz.)	3 or 4 T. cocoa plus 1 T. butter
cornstarch	1 tablespoon	2 T. flour or 2 tsp. quick-cooking tapioca
cracker crumbs	¾ cup	1 c. bread crumbs
dates	1 lb.	1½ c. dates, pitted and cut
dry mustard	1 teaspoon	1 T. prepared mustard
flour, self-rising	1 cup	1 c. all-purpose flour, ½ tsp. salt, and 1 tsp. baking powder
herbs, fresh	1 tablespoon	1 tsp. dried herbs
milk, sour	1 cup	1 T. lemon juice or vinegar plus sweet milk to make 1 c. (let stand 5 minutes)
milk, whole	1 cup	½ c. evaporated milk plus ½ cup water
min. marshmallows	10	1 lg. marshmallow
onion, fresh	1 small	1 T. instant minced onion, rehydrated
sugar, brown	½ cup	2 T. molasses in ½ c. granulated sugar
sugar, powdered	1 cup	1 c. granulated sugar plus 1 tsp. corn starch
tomato juice	1 cup	½ c. tomato sauce plus ½ c. water

When substituting cocoa for chocolate in cakes, the amount of flour must be reduced. Brown and white sugars usually can be interchanged.

Equivalency Chart

Food	Quantity	Yield
apple	1 medium	1 cup
banana, mashed	1 medium	⅓ cup
bread	1½ slices	1 cup soft crumbs
bread	1 slice	¼ cup fine, dry crumbs
butter	1 stick or ¼ pound	½ cup
cheese, American, cubed	1 pound	2⅔ cups
American grated	1 pound	5 cups
cream cheese	3-ounce package	6⅔ tablespoons
cocoa	1 pound-	4 cups
coconut	1½ pound package	2⅔ cups
cornmeal	1 pound	3 cups
cornstarch	1 pound	3 cups
egg	4-5 whole	1 cup
whites	8-10	1 cup
yolks	10-12	1 cup
evaporated milk	1 cup	3 cups whipped
flour, cake, sifted	1 pound	4½ cups
rye	1 pound	5 cups
white, sifted	1 pound	4 cups
white, unsifted	1 pound	3¾ cups
lemon	1 medium	3 tablespoons juice
noodles, cooked	8-ounce package	7 cups
uncooked	4 ounces (1½ cups)	2-3 cups cooked
macaroni, cooked	8-ounce package	6 cups
macaroni, uncooked	4 ounces (1¼ cups)	2¼ cups cooked
spaghetti, uncooked	7 ounces	4 cups cooked
nuts, chopped	¼ pound	1 cup
almonds	1 pound	3½ cups
walnuts, broken	1 pound	3 cups
walnuts, unshelled	1 pound	1½ to 1¾ cups
onion	1 medium	½ cup
orange	3-4 medium	1 cup juice
raisins	1 pound	3½ cups
rice, brown	1 cup	4 cups cooked
converted	1 cup	3½ cups cooked
regular	1 cup	3 cups cooked
wild	1 cup	4 cups cooked
sugar, brown	1 pound	2½ cups
powdered	1 pound	3½ cups
white	1 pound	2 cups

Some Nutrition Basics for a Healthier Life

Congratulations on choosing this cookbook full of great and fun chiropractic recipes.

And there's more – this special bonus article gives you the "why" and "how" of choosing health-friendly ingredients and food preparation methods.

Sometimes deciding what ingredients build health is easy (such as saying away from refined sugar, white flour and other "empty foods") and sometimes it's confusing.

After all, why choose between butter and margarine?

Just what is a trans fatty acid and why is it so bad for you?

Why invest in organic fruits and vegetables when conventionally grown produce is in every grocery store and is usually cheaper?

Why not enjoy the convenience of microwaved food?

Why does it seem as if you need an advanced degree in biochemistry to know how to shop and cook?

Organic or conventional?

Fruits, vegetables and other foods provide the human body with essential energy and nutrients to grow, work and play. Since most of us no longer grow our own foods, we rely on farmers. But, there is increasing evidence that not all tomatoes are alike. How a food is grown can affect its nutritional value and how good it is for us.

Nutritional content has been sacrificed by chemical applications of herbicides, pesticides and fertilizers.

No more earthworms

Soil fertility, crop selection and even the earthworms in the ground are needed to increase a crop's nutritional content.

Multiple chemical sprayings routinely applied to force larger and cheaper crop yields from the earth are destroying crop quality. It's possible to walk through a "conventional" field and see no earthworms in the soil.

Organic farmers produce crops that come from a more fertile soil, alive with the organisms needed for life's balance. Research shows that organically grown foods have more nutritional value – higher levels of vitamin C, magnesium, iron and phosphorus – and significantly reduced toxins such as nitrates.

On average, conventional produce has only 83% of the nutrients in organic produce. When our body has to use up its own minerals, energy and enzymes to digest foods with few minerals, energy and enzymes, we eventually get weak, sick, prematurely age and die before our time. Actually eating more of a less nutritious food may not even be the equivalent of eating less of a more nutritious food. It may be worse!

Chemical residues

In addition to the nutritional differences between organic and conventional farming, conventionally grown food is frequently tainted with chemical residues.

The pesticide sprays used to kill insects and reduce crop diseases are causing documented human health problems ranging from neurological conditions, depression, emotional and physical exhaustion, and a weakened immune system to cancer.

According to the Environmental Protection Agency (EPA), 60% of herbicides, 90% of fungicides and 30% of insecticides are known carcinogens (cancer causing). Pesticide residues are now detected in 50-95% of all U.S. foods.

Some fat-soluble pesticides have been added to animal feed to cut down on flies in the barnyard. The fecal matter became so toxic it ended up killing the flies! What about the pesticides that become part of the animal we eat?

While most U.S. foods tested for pesticide residues are found to be within the established legal limits, legal limits do not define safety. Washing and peeling foods like peaches, pears and apples can reduce the amount of exposure since pesticides tend to concentrate just on or under the skin of these fruits.

Unfortunately, for foods like squash, potatoes, spinach or green beans, the pesticides permeate the entire vegetable and cannot be washed off the skin. In these cases it may be best to consider buying organically grown foods.

Choosing organic foods over conventionally grown foods can be a wise choice for two reasons:

> One: you are protecting the environment from chemical pollution

> Two: you are protecting your body from chemical pollution

Organic farmers farm without the use of most conventional pesticides, synthetic fertilizers or sewage sludge. They feed and build the soil with natural fertilizers that reduce long-term environmental damage.

Instead of relying on synthetic sprays, organic farmers control crop diseases and destructive insects by relying on insect predators, physical barriers, crop rotation, tillage and hand weeding as well as cover crops and weed controlling mulches.

Consider joining the rising tide of consumers opting for organic foods and products. Organically grown foods are not only good for our health but also for our environment!

Sugar and Spice and Everything Nice

Table sugar (sucrose) used to be a natural substance from beets or cane but when refined into the white stuff all the vitamins and minerals are removed.

High fructose corn syrup is just as bad, in fact, many experts say it's far worse!

Where to get sweetness?

Gaining in popularity is the herb stevia, originally from Paraguay and used as a sweetener and flavor enhancer for centuries. Lo han fruit extract (SlimSweet™) and agave nectar are additional natural sweeteners.

Sugar alcohols can be considered artificial sweeteners although some like xylitol and sorbitol occur naturally in foods like fruits and berries. They do provide fewer calories than table sugar and despite the similar chemical structure to sugar are independent of insulin metabolism. Xylitol has been shown to dramatically reduce new tooth decay, to arrest and to provide some reversal of existing dental caries. The main drawbacks with the sugar alcohol sweeteners are that they may cause bloating, diarrhea and carbohydrate cravings.

There is no proof artificial sweeteners help you lose weight. So why use them? They may cause brain damage and cancer and other diseases. Wait, that's not a good reason to use them. What is? We don't know.

Saccharine (Sweet'NLow™) is the oldest artificial synthetic sweetener on the market and it isn't known for sure if it causes cancer.

Aspartame (NutraSweet™, Equal™) was originally banned by the FDA for its known toxicities. Approved under questionable political motives, it has been implicated in cancer, headaches, muscle pain and degeneration, and memory deterioration. Aspartame also suppresses the production of serotonin and makes you crave carbohydrates – this can make you gain weight!

Acesulfame (Sunette™, Sweet&Safe™, SweetOne™) is less well known and has some potential negative health effects of its own.

Splenda™ (sucralose) is not a natural sugar and affects the immune system by shrinking the thymus gland as well as potentially initiating anxiety, panic attacks, headaches, nerve pain, joint and chest pain, allergic type reactions and diarrhea.

Raw honey, organic maple syrup, evaporated cane juice, fruit juice, malt syrup from barley, rice syrup from barley and rice and date sugar from ground dates are all natural sugar sweeteners with beneficial nutrients not found in refined white sugar.

For low glycemic sweetening, enjoy the herb stevia, lo han fruit extract, agave nectar or even the natural sugar alcohol xylitol. Remember to find sweetness in life all the time and that sweetened foods should only be an occasional treat.

Fat. Good for you and bad for you. It depends...

Fats don't dissolve in water. Just pour oil (which is liquid fat) on water and you'll see two layers. They don't mix. Why is this important to you? Read on...

There are three kinds of fats: saturated, monounsaturated or polyunsaturated.

Saturated fats are found in animal and tropical oils. Monounsaturated fats include oils from olives and nuts. Polyunsaturated fats (or oils) are highly reactive oils that should not be heated for cooking.

At the turn of the century most dietary fatty acids were either saturated or monounsaturated, primarily from animal sources, coconut oil and olive oil.

You need fats

Saturated fats like those from butter actually play many essential roles in body chemistry. You need them to protect your cells and to absorb other fatty acids and minerals. Coconut oil is particularly abundant in easily digested medium chain fatty acids. These medium length saturated fatty acids can help maintain healthy cholesterol levels; support thyroid functioning;

support overall immune function by preventing bacterial, viral or fungal infections; and reduce symptoms of digestive disorders. Not only does coconut oil taste wonderful, it can help with weight loss and increase energy!

Olive oil, a monounsaturated oil, appears to lower the risk of coronary heart disease by lowering blood cholesterol levels. The antioxidant polyphenol in olive oil may prevent damage to blood vessels and cells by attacking free radicals that may be in our bodies. Olive oil also slows down acid overproduction in the digestive system and lowers the potential for ulcers and other GI issues.

While some fats are helpful like butter, coconut oil and olive oil, some fats are detrimental and not even all saturated fats are equal. For example, while both butter and margarine have saturated fats, butter is a natural food while margarine is not.

Margarine is artificially created from commercial vegetable oils by hydrogenation. Hydrogen is bubbled through the oils at high heat. This causes the molecules to change shape from a slightly bent into a stiffer trans formation hence the name trans fats.

There's one big problem with these synthetic stiff trans fats. They are toxic to humans. The fats dissolve into our cell membranes, causing the cells to leak.

Partially hydrogenated fats from vegetable oils actually block our ability to use essential fatty acids. This can result in sexual dysfunction, increased blood cholesterol and a weak immune system.

Despite the danger of hydrogenated oils they are widely used in the commercial food industry. Why? They're cheap. Also they don't spoil easily. You'll find them in doughnuts, crackers, cookies, pastries, deep-fat fried foods (yes, even 'fast food'), frostings and candies. They may be good for commercial foods' shelf life but they're not too good for your "shelf life."

Another very controversial oil that is heavily used in the commercial food industry is canola oil. Genetically engineered to reduce the content of toxic erucic acid, many studies suggest that canola oil is definitely not healthy for the cardiovascular system and may be associated with fibrotic lesions of the heart. Canola oil seems to deplete the body's store of vitamin E, retards growth and often contains trans fatty acids from deodorization or partial hydrogenation processes. Some researchers are concerned that the high level of easily oxidized polyunsaturated fats and low saturated fat level may cause the problems associated with canola oil in addition to the often high trans fatty acid levels from the oil's requisite refining before commercial use.

Want a healthier family? Enjoy the benefits of traditional oils and avoid hydrogenated oils and trans fatty acids. Consider serving organic butter or edible coconut oil to increase natural dietary saturated fat, extra virgin olive oil to enhance monounsaturated fat or drizzling expeller-expressed flax oil over salad to increase dietary polyunsaturated essential omega 3 fatty acids. Deciding between butter and margarine is simple – just say no to synthetic food – butter is better!

The pH secret to enjoying life

Chemists talk about the pH of things and discuss hydrogen. For everyone else however, pH is a measure of how much a substance is acid or alkaline. Most everything we eat is a little acidic (pH under 7) or alkaline (pH over 7) and can affect our body chemistry and our health. And, depending upon our body chemistry, an acid food may not always cause body acidity and an alkaline food may not always cause body alkalinity.

Research shows that a healthy person should be a little more alkaline than acid. In that state you have more energy and greater resistance to disease. An acidic person has less energy and may be courting trouble because many disease conditions thrive in an acidic environment.

That doesn't mean you can never eat acidic foods. As long as you have alkaline reserves to neutralize acids your body should have no trouble keeping the right pH balance for you. But if you're too acidic (hyperacid) your alkaline reserves are drained and your body systems are weakened.

Take care of your reserves, and your health, by eating a sufficient amount of alkaline-forming foods.

How to get it hot. Oven or microwave?

Most families no longer enjoy the benefits of Mom spending each day preparing the family dinner using whole foods and traditional food preparation methods. In our fast paced society today, home-cooked meals have been replaced to a large extent with instant food.

Processed food concerns aside, what are the health effects of preparing foods with a microwave oven instead of a conventional oven? After all, all cooked foods are equal, right? Well, maybe not!

Conventional ovens use heat to cook foods by heating from the outside-in using high temperatures. Microwaves, on the other hand, use low energy waves that penetrate foods through and through. The food absorbs the waves, vibrates at microscopic intensity and gets hot.

Microwaves, a form of radiation, are actually unhealthy radiation for people and pets. This radiation can leak throughout the whole kitchen when the microwave oven is being used.

Even the cockware frequently used for microwave cooking can also cause trouble since the plastics often used can leach plastic chemicals (phthalates) into food. These phthalates are associated with declining sperm counts, increase in sexual deformities, increase in testicular cancer and early puberty.

The most compelling evidence supporting the dangers of microwaves comes from a highly regarded study done by Swiss food scientist Dr. Hans Hertel. Dr. Hertel's startling findings indicated that eating microwaved food causes blood changes including increased cholesterol levels, elevated white blood cell counts, decreased red blood cells, production of bizarre compounds that are unknown in nature and decreased hemoglobin levels.

What can you do?

Some people have decided to put the microwave out of the house with the evening trash. Others have chosen to reduce microwave cooking to a bare minimum – briefly reheating leftovers (only in glass or non-plastic dishware).

Only you can decide what you do with new information, but remember that knowledge is power – make a powerful decision to choose health!

Selected References & Suggested Readings

Acid-Alkaline Balance. Retrieved from http://www.naturalhealthschool.com/acid-alkaline.html

Baroody TA. *Alkalize or Die.* Waynesville, NC: Holographic Health Press. 2002.

Do Environmental Chemicals Harm Humans? Retrieved from www.mercola.com/2004/march/6/environmental_chemicals.htm

Enig M, Fallon S. *Nourishing Traditions: The Cookbook that Challenges Politically Correct Nutrition and Diet Dictocrats.* 2nd Ed. Winona Lake, IN: New Trends Publishing, Inc. 2001:4-20.

Erasmus U. *Fats That Heal, Fats That Kill.* Burnaby, BC, Canada: Alive Books. 1986: 13-23,100-112.

Glimeny V. Artificial Sweeteners. *C & E News.* 2004:82(25):43. also available at:pubs.acs.org/cen/whatstuff/stuff/8225sweeteners.html

Holden D. (Ed.) *The Hazards of Microwave Cooked Food.* Retrieved from www.osiris.org.nz/Articles/MicrowaveFoodHazards.htm

How to Avoid the Top 10 Most Common Toxins. Retrieved from www.mercola.com/2005/feb/19/common_toxins.htm

Neustaedter R. *Sugar/Sweeteners.* Retrieved from www.cure-guide.com/Natural_Health_Newsletter/Sugar_Sweeteners/sugar_sweeteners.html

Phthalates. Retrieved from www.ijc.org/rel/boards/hptf/hptfnews/vol3is4e.html

Wilson G. *Agriculture and Nutrition.* Retrieved from www.westonaprice.org/farming/agriculture-nutrition.html

www.ams.usda.gov/nop/Consumers/brochure.html

www.coconutoil-online.com/coconut_info_links.html

www.foodnews.org

www.holisticmed.com/sweet/#guide